Contents

Praise

"Most people with type 2 diabetes do not struggle because they lack discipline. They struggle because nobody explains what is actually happening. I am a senior, and for years I thought my diabetes had simply gone too far and that getting fatter was just the price of staying alive on medication. My numbers would improve, but my body felt worse, and no doctor ever explained why. This book shocked me in the best way. It made me realize that forcing sugar into already overfilled cells can make the underlying problem worse, even if the lab work looks better. For the first time, I understood the root cause and felt like I had a real path to regain control."

— Robert H., Retired Teacher, Type 2 Diabetes Patient

"As a registered dietitian nutritionist, I see people overwhelmed by rules that do not connect to real physiology. This book removes that confusion by explaining insulin resistance as an overflow problem and then tying every recommendation back to that mechanism. The benefits are clear and practical: reduce the constant sugar input, lower insulin demand, support loss of visceral fat, and improve post-meal stability without extreme restriction. I was surprised by how well it links waist circumference and fatty liver risk to what patients can actually do week to week."

— Nadia L., Registered Dietitian Nutritionist (RDN)

"As a primary care physician, I am always looking for resources that help patients understand the why, not just the what. This book does that while staying balanced. It is not anti-medicine. It is pro-root-cause, and it clearly explains why treating glucose numbers without addressing diet and fuel storage can lead to a slow worsening path. I especially appreciate the careful warning that fasting requires smart medication adjustments for anyone on insulin or sulfonylureas. The section on fatty liver showing up early was genuinely eye-opening and will change how I talk to patients."

— Anika R., MD

"As a diabetes educator, I have never seen insulin resistance explained this clearly for everyday readers. The hallway and storage rooms metaphor makes it easy for someone to understand what is happening inside their body without shame. The book also gives a refreshing reframe: it is not just about eating less, it is about changing signals and restoring flexibility. I was surprised by how helpful the discussion of adaptive thermogenesis is, because it explains why people plateau and regain even when they are trying hard."

— Marcus J., Certified Diabetes Care and Education Specialist (CDCES)

"I have read plenty of diabetes advice that turns into carb wars or perfection pressure. This book felt different because it focuses on what actually drives the problem in modern life: added sugar, refined starch, constant snacking, and ultra-processed foods. The benefit for me was clarity. I finally understood why whole-food carbs are not the same as sugar and flour, and why my waist matters more than the scale. I was honestly surprised at how quickly my fear dropped once the disease made sense."

— Simone K., Type 2 Diabetes Patient

"As a bariatric support coach, I appreciate how this book talks about surgery without hype. It explains that remission after surgery is not magic, it is a system shift involving hormones, appetite, and fuel handling, and it acknowledges that long-term behavior support still matters. That message helps readers who are scared or discouraged realize the bigger benefit: the body is changeable. The story about remission returning over time was a powerful reminder, and it made the lifestyle strategy in this book feel even more important and more achievable."

— Daniel S., Bariatric Support Coach and Patient Advocate

Disclaimer and Legal Notice

Introduction to The Diabetes Type 2 Reset

I n **1980**, type 2 diabetes was still relatively rare on a global scale. Today, it's everywhere. The World Health Organization reported that the number of adults living with diabetes has **almost quadrupled since 1980**, reaching **422 million** (World Health Organization, 2016). That is not a slow genetic drift. That is a rapid environmental shift.

So here's the question that should make you pause:

What changed so fast in one generation that millions of bodies could not keep up?

It wasn't your DNA.

It was the food.

The uncomfortable truth nobody says out loud

Type 2 diabetes is mostly a dietary disease.

Not a "you're broken forever" disease. Not a "bad luck" disease. Not a "your pancreas randomly gave up" disease.

And if it's mostly caused by what we eat, then the most hopeful idea becomes possible:

Type 2 diabetes is often reversible.

That's **Fact #1**.

Fact #2 is darker: **most conventionally treated patients gradually get worse**, needing more meds and often eventually insulin, because the usual approach focuses on "lowering blood sugar numbers" without fixing why the sugar is high in the first place (American Diabetes Association, 2025; Bagust & Beale,

2003).

This book is here to change that story.

If you've been told the only way to improve type 2 is with a strict, pricey, joyless diet, I want to reassure you: there's another way.

You can eat meals that are **quick, comforting, and flavorful** while working towards better blood sugar.

That's exactly what I wrote in my other book, *The 5-Ingredient Diabetic Diet Cookbook for Beginners*. A **60-day meal plan** with **simple recipes** you can make in about **30 minutes a day**, using affordable ingredients.

Here is the title to search on Amazon:

The 5 Ingredient Diabetic Diet Cookbook for Beginners:

How to Stabilize Blood Sugar in Just 30 Minutes a Day - 60 Days of Simple, Delicious Type 2 Diabetes Meal Plans Under 10$

Scan this code to be taken there directly:

SCAN ME

What's actually happening inside your body

Most people are taught a simple explanation:

"Your blood sugar is high. You need medicine to push it down."

But that explanation skips the most important part.

The overflow problem

Think of your body like a set of storage rooms.

- Your **blood** is the hallway.
- Your **cells** are the rooms.
- **Glucose** is the stuff being delivered.
- **Insulin** is the key that opens the doors so glucose can move from the hallway into the rooms.

In type 2 diabetes, the problem is not that insulin "forgot how to work."

The deeper problem is that **the rooms are already stuffed**.

When your cells are overflowing with stored fuel, they resist taking more. Blood sugar rises because the hallway gets jammed with glucose that has nowhere to go.

So what do many treatments do?

They give you more insulin, or drugs that increase insulin, to force more glucose into already packed cells.

It can improve the blood test, but it can worsen the overflow.

That's why insulin can be a trap for many people with type 2: it often lowers glucose but is also linked with **weight gain** in many real-world cases, which can fuel the underlying problem (Pontiroli et al., 2011; McFarlane, 2009).

This is why diabetes can feel like quicksand: the harder you push in the wrong direction, the deeper you sink.

Why "eat less, move more" often fails

You've heard it a thousand times:

"Just cut calories."

But your body is not a calculator. It's a survival machine.

When calories drop, the body can respond by lowering energy expenditure, a phenomenon often called **adaptive thermogenesis**. In plain language: your body can **burn fewer calories than expected**, making weight loss slower and regain easier (Most et al., 2020; Müller et al., 2015).

So if someone says, "Calories are all that matters," ask them:

Then why does the body change how many calories it burns when you diet?

A better lens is this:

Obesity and type 2 diabetes are strongly hormonal

Insulin is a major fat-storage hormone. If insulin stays high all day, every day, your body is being signaled to store, not burn.

That's why this book isn't just about "eating less."

It's about changing the signals.

The liver connection nobody checks early enough

Here's a pattern that shows up again and again:

Fatty liver often comes before type 2 diabetes.

Non-alcoholic fatty liver disease (NAFLD) is strongly linked to insulin resistance, and research shows NAFLD can predict future risk of type 2 diabetes (Ming et al., 2015).

So if your liver is storing excess fat, it's like a clogged filter in your metabolism. The system backs up.

Fructose makes this worse

Fructose (especially from added sugars like high fructose corn syrup) is handled differently than glucose. A large body of research links high fructose intake to increased liver fat and increased **de novo lipogenesis**, which is your liver turning sugar into fat (Softic et al., 2016; Stanhope et al., 2009).

That matters because it explains something people argue about nonstop:

"Is saturated fat the villain?"

Blood saturated fat levels are not only about what you eat. They're also shaped by what your liver *makes* when sugar intake is high and the liver shifts into a fat-producing mode (Volk et al., 2014; Bajahzer et al., 2022).

So the conversation is not as simple as "fat bad, carbs good" or "carbs bad, fat good."

The real enemy is the modern combo:

- **added sugar**
- **refined starch**
- **constant snacking**
- **ultra-processed foods**

That's where the epidemic lives.

Why your waist matters more than the scale

If you want one easy body clue that correlates strongly with diabetes risk, it's not your weight. It's your **waist**.

Large studies show waist circumference is strongly associated with future risk of type 2 diabetes, even beyond overall body fat (Jayedi et al., 2022).

Why?

Because **visceral fat**, the deep belly fat around organs, is metabolically active and strongly tied to insulin resistance, more so than subcutaneous fat (the pinchable fat under the skin) (Xu et al., 2024).

So we're not just trying to "lose weight."

We're trying to lose **the dangerous kind**.

The clue hiding in plain sight: real-world diet evidence

If carbs automatically caused diabetes, then every high-carb culture would be diabetic.

But that's not what we see.

Kitava: high carb, low diabetes signals

Traditional Kitavans ate a high-carbohydrate diet built around whole foods, not ultra-processed sugar and flour. Researchers found markedly different insulin patterns compared with Western controls (Lindeberg et al., 1999).

That doesn't mean "carbs are magic."

It means **food quality and processing matter**, and constant added sugar is not the same as traditional whole-food carbs.

Mediterranean pattern: proven heart protection

The Mediterranean diet pattern has some of the strongest evidence in nutrition science for cardiovascular protection. The PREDIMED trial reported fewer major cardiovascular events in Mediterranean diet groups compared with a control diet (Estruch et al., 2013/2018).

And since heart disease is the number one killer of people with type 2, this matters.

What actually helps, in one sentence

There are **two core moves** that work together:

1. **Put less sugar in.**
2. **Burn the stored sugar.**

That is the foundation.

And this is where fasting enters the story.

Fasting isn't new. It's old medicine

Long before modern diabetes drugs, doctors used fasting and periods of undernutrition as a tool in diabetes care. Historical medical literature discusses fasting-based approaches in the pre-insulin era (Mazur, 2011).

You're not doing something trendy.

You're using a tool humans have used for a very long time: **intermittency**.

Modern research reviews suggest intermittent fasting can improve glycemic control and weight in many people with type 2 diabetes, especially when medications are properly managed to prevent hypoglycemia (Sharma et al., 2023).

Important note: if you use insulin or sulfonylureas, fasting can drop glucose fast. That is not dangerous if handled correctly, but it **does require smart medication adjustments**.

Surgery proves a powerful point (even if you never want surgery)

Bariatric surgery helps many people achieve remission, and strong trials show it can prevent or delay type 2 diabetes in high-risk groups (Carlsson et al., 2012).

But surgery is not "magic stomach shrinking."

It changes hormones, appetite signaling, and how the body handles fuel.

Which proves something huge:

The system is changeable.

And if the body can shift that much through surgery, the right lifestyle strategy can shift it too, without scalpels.

Leigh Ann, age 40 chose **Roux-en-Y bariatric surgery** believing it would be her lasting solution to diabetes, and at first it worked. Her weight dropped, blood sugars normalized, and her A1c went into remission. Over time, stress and old habits resurfaced, and eating around the pouch slowly stretched it, bringing hunger back and eventually her diabetes as well. Now she manages not only rising blood sugars again, but also **lifelong nutrition deficiencies** that require constant monitoring and supplements. Her story is a quiet reminder that **bariatric surgery is not always the solution**. It can be a powerful tool, but without long-term support, behavior change, and compassion, remission can be temporary and the journey far more complex than promised.

Cure vs. control: the line this book draws

Moves that can drive remission for many people (when done correctly):

- Meaningful, sustained weight loss (Lean et al., 2018; Lean et al., 2019)
- Carbohydrate reduction for many people (Goldenberg et al., 2021)
- Intermittent fasting (Sharma et al., 2023)
- Bariatric surgery (Carlsson et al., 2012)

Moves that often control numbers without fixing the overflow:

- More and more insulin without addressing diet (McFarlane, 2009)
- Drug stacking while lifestyle stays the same (American Diabetes Association, 2025)

This book is not anti-medicine.

It's pro-root-cause.

What you're going to do in this book

You're going to follow a **doctor-free, real-life 7-step system** designed to:

- lower blood sugar
- reduce visceral fat
- calm insulin resistance
- restore metabolic flexibility
- and help you feel like you're in control again

No obsession. No starvation. No fake perfection.

Just the exact levers that matter.

Because when you finally understand the disease, you stop fearing it.

And you start reversing it.

In the next step you will find the first action that makes everything else easier: how to stop feeding the overflow without living on sadness and salad.

STEP 1 — Understand America's #1 Dietary Epidemic

The Epidemic Isn't Random

Here's an uplifting fact to start with: **Type 2 diabetes can go into remission** for many people, meaning blood sugar returns below the diabetes range for at least three months without glucose-lowering meds, as defined by an international expert consensus. (Riddle et al., 2021; American Diabetes Association, 2021). That is not a hype claim. It is a medical definition.

Now the hard part.

In 2016, the World Health Organization dropped a headline that should have stopped the world for a minute: **the number of adults living with diabetes almost quadrupled since 1980**, reaching **422 million** by 2014 (World Health Organization, 2016). One generation. Not a slow drift across centuries. A sharp, modern spike.

So ask the obvious question: **What changed?**

Because genes do not rewrite themselves in 40 years.

Two facts about Type 2 (read these twice)

Fact #1: Remission is possible.

In the DiRECT clinical trial (run in real primary care clinics), **46%** of people in the intensive weight-management program reached remission at 1 year (Lean et al., 2018). That is almost half.

Fact #2: The "usual" path is progression.

Traditional care often treats Type 2 like a one-way street: more meds over time, sometimes insulin later. The UK Prospective Diabetes Study described Type 2 as a **progressive disease**, with blood sugar control worsening over years alongside declining beta-cell function (UKPDS Group, 1995). That is the story most people get told.

This book exists because those two facts collide.

If remission can happen, and progression is common, then the real question is: **what decides which track you end up on?**

A disease older than pyramids, but not like this

Diabetes is not new. Ancient medical writings described people who were intensely thirsty, peeing constantly, and wasting away. Thousands of years ago, doctors noticed something eerie: urine that tasted sweet, and ants that seemed weirdly interested in it (Karamanou et al., 2016). That "melting away" picture is what we now recognize as untreated Type 1 diabetes.

For most of human history, diabetes was rare and usually deadly.

Then insulin was discovered and purified in the early 1920s, and it was like watching someone pull a person back from the edge. Kids who were fading fast could suddenly gain weight, wake up, and live (World Health Organization, 2016). It was one of medicine's greatest wins.

But here's the twist: **insulin did not end the diabetes story.** It changed it.

As doctors paid attention, they realized not all diabetes looked the same. Some people had little or no insulin. Others had insulin, sometimes plenty of it, but their body acted like it could not "hear" the message. That difference was recognized as early as the 1930s in the medical literature on insulin sensitivity

(Himsworth, 1936/2013).

That second pattern is what dominates today.

Type 2 is now the main driver of the epidemic. And epidemics are rarely random.

The rise that genetics can't explain

The WHO's timeline is the cleanest alarm bell: almost quadrupling since 1980 (World Health Organization, 2016). When you see a curve that steep, you should think "environment," not "destiny."

Yes, family history matters. But genetics is like the blueprint of a building. The blueprint does not change overnight. The neighborhood does.

So what changed after about 1980?

It was not just "people got lazy." That story is too simple, and honestly, it is cruel. People did not suddenly lose their willpower in the same decade all over the globe.

What changed was the **food environment** and the way eating got woven into daily life: what's available, what's cheap, what's marketed, and how often we eat without even calling it eating.

A simple timeline: what changed after ~1980?

Before 1980:

- Fewer ultra-processed foods as the default
- Less constant snacking culture
- Meals were more clearly "meals"

Around 1977 to 1980:

- National nutrition messaging shifts toward higher carbohydrate intake and lower fat intake (U.S. Dietary Guidelines for Americans, 1980; U.S. Senate Select Committee on Nutrition and Human Needs, 1977/1978)

1980s to 2000s:

- "Low-fat" becomes a marketing superpower
- Refined carbs and added sugars fill the taste gap
- Portions expand, and snacks become normal meals

By the 2000s:

- Ultra-processed foods and sugary drinks are everywhere
- Eating occasions rise, and the time between eating shrinks (Piernas & Popkin, 2010)

That is not nostalgia. That is a behavioral shift documented in research. U.S. adults increased snacking occasions from 1977 to 2006, and snacks grew as a share of daily calories (Piernas & Popkin, 2010). More eating opportunities means more glucose spikes, more insulin calls, more "storage mode" signals.

And it is not just how often we eat. It is what we are eating.

In a tightly controlled NIH study, people ate a diet of ultra-processed foods or a diet of minimally processed foods. The meals were designed to match on key nutrients like macros, sugar, sodium, and fiber. Yet on the ultra-processed diet, participants ate more calories and gained weight in just two weeks (Hall et al., 2019). That is wild. It suggests the modern food environment can push your body toward overeating even when the nutrition label looks similar.

And there is more: observational research links higher ultra-processed food intake to higher Type 2 diabetes risk (Srour et al., 2020). Observational studies do not prove cause alone, but when you combine them with controlled experiments like Hall's trial, the pattern gets harder to ignore.

The "dietary" argument, said carefully

Let's be precise: Type 2 diabetes is not caused by one single food. It is not "you ate one donut and now you're broken."

It is better described like this:

Type 2 happens when your body is forced to live in a high-insulin, high-fuel environment for too long.

That environment is heavily shaped by diet, especially:

- **Refined carbohydrates** that digest fast and spike glucose
- **Sugary drinks** that deliver sugar with almost no fullness
- **Ultra-processed foods** engineered for maximum repeat-bite
- **Constant eating** that never lets insulin fully come down

You do not need to be a scientist to get the logic. If your bloodstream is a highway, your blood sugar is traffic. Insulin is the traffic cop. When traffic surges all day long, the cop is constantly shouting orders. Eventually, cells stop listening. That is insulin resistance in plain language.

Sugary drinks are a perfect example because they are easy to measure. Meta-analyses have found that higher sugar-sweetened beverage intake is associated with higher Type 2 diabetes risk (Imamura et al., 2015; Wang et al., 2014). Again, that does not mean one soda equals diabetes. It means the trend points in one direction: a daily habit matters.

This is why the epidemic has a "diet-driven environment" feel. Not blame. Not moral failure. Environment.

The hidden cost: when chronic disease becomes "normal"

Here is the scary part, and the motivating part.

When something becomes common, people stop treating it like a crisis.

Prediabetes becomes a shrug. High A1C becomes "kinda normal for your age." Being tired all the time becomes "life." Needing three medications by 45 becomes "adulting."

But diabetes is not just a blood sugar number. It is a body-wide stressor. It stacks risk on risk.

It is also expensive in a way most people do not feel until it hits them.

In the United States, the estimated cost of diagnosed diabetes was **$245 billion** in 2012 (American Diabetes Association, 2013). And by 2022, estimates rose to **$412.9 billion**, with diabetes care accounting for about **1 in 4** health care dollars, according to the analysis (Parker et al., 2024). Those are not abstract numbers. That is insurance premiums, hospital systems, missed work, caregiver burnout, and families quietly rearranging life around a chronic condition.

And that is just money.

The bigger cost is the slow theft: energy, confidence, mobility, eyesight, kidney function, and the feeling that your body is "betraying" you.

This book is going to flip that story.

Because your body is not failing. **Your body is responding to the environment.**

Actionable: your self-audit (no shame, just signal)

You cannot change what you will not name. So this chapter ends with a simple inventory. Not to diagnose you. To help you see your starting point clearly.

Risk signals (check any that apply):

- Waist size climbing over the last few years
- Blood pressure trending up
- Triglycerides high and HDL low (a common metabolic pattern)
- Family history of Type 2 diabetes
- History of gestational diabetes or PCOS
- Sleep is short or poor most nights
- You feel "hangry," shaky, or moody when meals are delayed
- You crave carbs or sweets in a way that feels automatic

Symptom inventory (these can be subtle):

- You are thirsty a lot
- You pee more than you used to, especially at night
- You crash hard after meals
- Your vision gets blurry sometimes

- Cuts heal slowly
- You get frequent infections (skin, gums, urinary)
- You feel brain fog, especially in the afternoon

If you checked several, do not panic. Treat it like a dashboard light. It is information.

Actionable: your starting line labs and numbers

You deserve a clear baseline. If you have access to a clinician, ask for these. If you already have a diagnosis, ask anyway so you can track progress.
   Core glucose markers:

- **HbA1c** (3-month average blood sugar)
- **Fasting glucose**
- Optional but useful: **fasting insulin** or **C-peptide** (helps explain insulin output vs resistance)

Metabolic health markers:

- **Lipid panel** (especially triglycerides and HDL)
- **Blood pressure**
- **Waist circumference** (measure at the level of your belly button, relaxed)
- **Weight** plus an honest note on where you store fat (central belly fat matters)

Organ and complication screening:

- **Kidneys:** creatinine/eGFR, and urine albumin-to-creatinine ratio
- **Liver:** ALT and AST (fatty liver often travels with insulin resistance)

One more safety note that matters: **If you are on insulin or medications that can cause low blood sugar, changing food fast can change your medication**

needs fast. Always coordinate dose changes with a qualified clinician. (We will talk about this more in Step 1, Chapter 2 and Step 2.)

Where this is going next

If Type 2 is not random, and the environment is a major driver, then the next problem is huge:

How do you treat the right problem?

Because Type 1 and Type 2 are often talked about like they are the same thing with different severity. They are not. And if you confuse them, you end up chasing numbers instead of fixing the cause.

In the next chapter, we are going to separate Type 1 vs Type 2 so clearly that you will never mix them up again, and you will understand why "just add insulin" is often the wrong story for Type 2.

Type 1 or 2?

Uplifting fact first: **getting the diabetes type right can change everything**. It changes which tools work, which ones backfire, and what "better" even means. Mislabeling is not just a paperwork problem. It can be a safety problem.

Diabetes mellitus is a group of conditions where **blood glucose stays too high**. High glucose can cause the classic symptoms most people have heard about: intense thirst, peeing a lot, fatigue, blurry vision, and unexplained weight loss. When glucose rises high enough, it spills into urine and drags water with it, like a leak that will not stop. The body gets dehydrated and stressed. (American Diabetes Association, 2025). (Diabetes Journals)

But here's the key idea for this chapter:

Type 1 and Type 2 can share the same symptom, high blood sugar, while having totally different root problems.

If you treat the symptom but ignore the root, you can end up stuck on the "more meds forever" treadmill.

The simplest way to understand it

Think of blood sugar like fuel in your bloodstream.

- **Insulin is the key** that unlocks your cells so fuel can get in.
- **Type 1** is mainly a problem of **not enough keys**.
- **Type 2** is mainly a problem of **sticky locks**.

Same fuel. Different failure.

Type 1: the missing-insulin problem

Type 1 diabetes is usually autoimmune (or can be caused from surgical removal of all or part of the pancreas). The immune system slowly attacks the insulin-making beta cells in the pancreas. Over time, insulin production drops until it is not enough to keep glucose controlled. That is why Type 1 often shows up suddenly, sometimes with dramatic symptoms. (Donath et al., 2022). (PubMed Central)

This is also why **insulin is not optional** in Type 1. It is replacement therapy, like glasses for vision or a cast for a broken bone.

Type 2: the insulin-resistance problem

Type 2 diabetes usually starts with **insulin resistance**. The body still makes insulin, sometimes a lot of it, but the cells respond poorly. So the pancreas pushes out more insulin to force glucose into the cells. That can work for a while. Then the system gets overwhelmed and blood sugar rises. That is why Type 2 often sneaks in quietly and is found on routine labs. (American Diabetes Association, 2025). (Diabetes Journals)

This is why Type 2 is not just "a little Type 1." It is a different problem with a different strategy.

Why confusion happens

Because both types can show high A1C and high glucose.
Many people assume:

· "High blood sugar means I need more insulin."

That is sometimes true, especially in Type 1. But in Type 2, the deeper issue is often that the body is already swimming in insulin signals, and cells have learned to ignore them.

If you only chase the glucose number, you can improve the lab while the underlying system keeps getting worse.

This is one reason Type 2 is often called progressive in conventional care. Over time, more medication is typically needed to keep glucose controlled. The body's ability to handle the overload keeps declining. (That does not mean you are doomed. It means the default approach often does not address the driver.) (American Diabetes Association, 2025). (Diabetes Journals)

The emergency differences you must know

Most day-to-day symptoms overlap, but the dangerous "crisis" patterns differ.

Type 1 can lead to diabetic ketoacidosis (DKA).

When insulin is very low, the body cannot use glucose well and starts breaking down fat rapidly, producing ketones and acid. DKA can become life-threatening fast. The warning signs can include deep rapid breathing, severe nausea, vomiting and/or belly pain, confusion, and fruity-smelling breath. This is an emergency. (Hamman et al., 2014). (PubMed Central)

Type 2 can lead to hyperosmolar hyperglycemic state (HHS).

This is more about extremely high glucose and severe dehydration.Often associated with an underlying infection or illness. It can cause seizures, confusion, and coma. It is also an emergency.

If you ever suspect DKA or HHS, that is not a "wait and see" situation.

The one-page compare chart

Actionable: "Which type do I likely have?" discussion points

This is not a self-diagnosis checklist. It is a conversation starter to bring to a clinician.

Ask about:

- **Age and speed of onset:** Did symptoms hit fast, over days or weeks, or slowly over years?
- **Weight change:** Was there rapid unexplained weight loss?
- **Family and autoimmune history:** Any thyroid disease, celiac disease, vitiligo, or other autoimmune conditions?
- **Labs that can help clarify:**
- **C-peptide** (how much insulin your body is producing)
- **Islet autoantibodies** (markers that support autoimmune Type 1 patterns)
- A1C and glucose patterns over time (American Diabetes Association, 2025). (Diabetes Journals)

And if you were told "Type 2" but you are lean, symptoms came on fast, or you had DKA, it is worth asking about whether you could have an autoimmune form.

Actionable: know the diagnosis numbers

These are commonly used ADA thresholds:

- **A1C:** diabetes at **6.5% or higher**
- **Fasting plasma glucose:** diabetes at **126 mg/dL (7.0 mmol/L) or higher**
- **2-hour OGTT:** diabetes at **200 mg/dL (11.1 mmol/L) or higher**
- **Random glucose: 200 mg/dL (11.1 mmol/L) or higher** plus classic symptoms (American Diabetes Association, n.d.; American Diabetes Association, 2025). (American Diabetes Association)

Med safety warning you cannot skip

If you are taking insulin or medications that can cause hypoglycemia, changing food patterns can change medication needs quickly.

If you lower carbs, skip meals, or start fasting while on certain diabetes meds, your blood sugar can drop too low. That can be dangerous.

So the rule is simple: **food changes and med changes often need to be coordinated.** Do not "tough it out" through frequent lows. Bring the data to your prescriber and adjust safely.

The big mistake: treating Type 2 like Type 1

Here is the mindset shift this book is built on:

- In Type 1, insulin is the missing piece.
- In Type 2, insulin is often already high, and the real goal is to reduce resistance and overload.

That is why a "just add more insulin" mindset can manage the number while leaving the cause untouched. It is not that insulin is evil. It is that insulin is not the full answer for Type 2.

And this matters emotionally, too.

If you think Type 2 is just bad luck, you may feel powerless. If you understand it as a mismatch between your biology and a modern food environment, you can start making moves that actually change the game.

Coming next

Now that you can separate Type 1 from Type 2, we're going to widen the camera lens.

Because diabetes is not only about glucose.

In the next chapter, you'll see how insulin resistance and chronic high blood sugar ripple through the whole body: heart, liver, brain, hormones, nerves, and energy. And once you see that, you will stop thinking, "I just need a better A1C," and start thinking, "I want my whole body back."

Collateral Damage

When blood sugar improves, the risk of "small-vessel" damage to eyes and kidneys drops too. In the UKPDS follow-up, earlier better glucose control showed a meaningful reduction in microvascular complications over time. (New England Journal of Medicine)

Now the truth most people never get told on day one:

Diabetes is not a "sugar-only" disease. It is a whole-body disease.

It can touch your eyes, kidneys, nerves, heart, brain, liver, skin, hormones, and even how well wounds heal. It is like having one problem in the bloodstream that sends ripples into every room of the house.

If you only focus on the glucose number, you might miss what is actually happening underneath.

Microvascular vs macrovascular

Think of your blood vessels like roads.

- **Microvascular complications** happen in the tiny roads, the narrow side streets that deliver oxygen to delicate tissues.
- **Macrovascular complications** happen in the highways, the big pipes that feed the heart, brain, and legs.

Both matter. Both can change your life.

The microvascular hit list

Eyes: retinopathy and vision loss

The retina is the light-sensitive layer at the back of your eye. It needs a steady, gentle blood supply. Diabetes can weaken those tiny retinal vessels so they leak. Then the eye tries to "fix" the problem by growing new vessels, but the new ones are fragile. They bleed easily. Scar tissue can form. Vision can blur, then fade.

Diabetic retinopathy is widely described as **a leading cause of blindness in working-age adults**, and the scariest part is that early damage can have no obvious symptoms. (American Diabetes Association)

The emotional part nobody says out loud: losing vision does not just steal sight. It steals independence. Driving. Reading. Seeing faces clearly. Even feeling safe walking down stairs.

Action you can take: a yearly dilated eye exam or retinal imaging is not "extra." It is protective. (American Diabetes Association)

Kidneys: nephropathy and kidney failure

Your kidneys are high-powered filters. They clean your blood all day, every day. Diabetes can damage the tiny filtering units. Early on, you might not feel anything. Later, protein can leak into urine. Then filtration drops. Toxins build up. Energy collapses. Appetite disappears. Swelling can show up in ankles and around eyes.

In the U.S., **diabetes is a major cause of end-stage kidney disease**, and the CDC continues to highlight diabetes as a leading driver of kidney failure requiring dialysis or transplant. (CDC)

Dialysis is not a mild inconvenience. It is hours of life every week attached to a machine, planning everything around treatment days. That is why kidney protection is a core goal of your reset.

Action you can take: ask for:

- Urine albumin-to-creatinine ratio (early "leak" check)
- eGFR and creatinine (filter function check)

Those two tests can catch trouble early.

Nerves: neuropathy and the "silent injury" trap

Diabetic nerve damage can feel like tingling, burning, numbness, or electric pain, usually starting in the feet. Some people describe it like walking on hot sand, or like socks made of pins. Others feel nothing at all, which sounds lucky until you realize what pain is for.

Pain is an alarm system. When it is broken, injuries can happen without you noticing. A small blister becomes a wound. A wound becomes an ulcer. Infection sneaks in.

Reviews commonly describe diabetic peripheral neuropathy as affecting a large portion of people with diabetes, with prevalence varying by age and duration. (PubMed Central)

Action you can take: a simple foot routine:

- Look at your feet daily (top, bottom, between toes)
- Feel for hot spots, swelling, or cuts
- Wear shoes that fit and do not rub
- Report numbness, burning, or non-healing sores early

The macrovascular hit list

Macrovascular complications are the big, headline events: heart attacks, strokes, circulation loss in legs. These are largely driven by atherosclerosis, where arteries become damaged and inflamed over time and plaque builds inside the vessel wall.

Heart disease

Diabetes is strongly associated with higher cardiovascular risk. Classic epidemiology from the Framingham Heart Study and later summaries describe diabetes as linked with roughly a **2 to 4 times higher risk** of major cardiovascular events compared with people without diabetes. (PubMed Central)

This is why some people with Type 2 feel fine, then suddenly have a heart attack as their "first symptom." Diabetes can be quiet until it is not.

Stroke

A stroke is a blood flow failure in the brain, often due to blocked arteries or clots. Diabetes increases stroke risk and worsens outcomes. The brain is unforgiving about oxygen shortages.

Peripheral artery disease and amputations

When blood flow to the legs and feet drops, walking can hurt. Skin can heal slowly. A tiny cut can turn into a chronic wound.

The CDC describes how diabetes complications like poor circulation and nerve damage raise the risk of **lower-limb amputation**, and CDC reporting has long noted diabetes as a leading cause of nontraumatic lower-extremity amputations. (CDC)

That is the nightmare scenario. But it is also one of the clearest reasons to treat diabetes as whole-body care, not just a glucose number.

The "other complications" that deserve attention

Diabetes also connects to conditions that do not fit neatly into "small vessel" or "big vessel" categories.

Fatty liver: the overlooked middleman

Fatty liver disease has been renamed by many experts as **MASLD** (metabolic dysfunction-associated steatotic liver disease), but you will still hear NAFLD everywhere. It means too much fat stored in liver cells.

Recent reviews estimate fatty liver affects **around 70% of people with Type 2 diabetes**. (PubMed Central)

And global prevalence in adults is often summarized as around **30%**. (PubMed)

This matters because the liver is a major glucose and fat traffic controller. When the liver is stuffed with fat, insulin resistance tends to worsen. We will go deep on this later, because it is one of the most important "hidden engines" in Type 2.

Infections: when sugar becomes fuel for germs

People with diabetes have a higher risk of infections, with reviews describing roughly **1.5 to 4-fold increased risk**, especially for serious infections like kidney and foot infections. (PubMed Central)

If you have frequent UTIs, skin infections, fungal infections, or slow-healing wounds, that is not random bad luck. It can be a metabolic signal.

PCOS, fertility, and hormone chaos

Polycystic ovary syndrome (PCOS) is tightly linked to insulin resistance and higher long-term risk of dysglycemia and Type 2 diabetes. (ScienceDirect)

This is one reason the "blood sugar only" story is too small. Insulin resistance can show up as acne, irregular cycles, unwanted hair growth, and fertility struggles. That is not vanity. That is physiology.

Brain health: the "Type 3 diabetes" idea

Some researchers use the phrase "Type 3 diabetes" to describe insulin resistance patterns in the brain that may overlap with Alzheimer's disease. The relationship is complex, but evidence supports Type 2 diabetes as a risk factor for cognitive decline and Alzheimer's disease in epidemiologic research and meta-analyses. (PubMed Central)

You do not need to panic about this. You need to understand the direction of the risk: metabolic health matters for brain health.

Cancer risk

Large analyses suggest Type 2 diabetes is associated with higher risk for several cancers, with some evidence supporting causal links for certain types such as liver, pancreatic, and endometrial cancer. (Diabetes Journals)

Again, diabetes is not a "number problem." It is a whole-body environment problem.

The part that changes everything

Here is the line that will guide the rest of this book:

Treat the cause, not the symptom.

Lowering glucose matters, especially for preventing microvascular damage. (PubMed)

But focusing only on glucose can be incomplete, and in some intensive strategies, very aggressive glucose lowering has not consistently translated into better cardiovascular outcomes and has even shown harm in certain trial settings. (New England Journal of Medicine)

So what is the deeper cause in Type 2?

This is where Step 2 begins to peek around the corner.

Type 2 diabetes is strongly connected to **insulin resistance**, and often **high insulin levels** for years before diagnosis. Blood sugar is the smoke. Insulin resistance is the fire.

Callout: Your body is not failing. You are responding to the environment.

Actionables: "Beyond glucose" tracking list

Starting today, track more than sugar. Pick 3 to start and build from there:

- **Waist size** (monthly): belly fat is a strong insulin resistance signal
- **Blood pressure** (weekly)
- **Triglycerides and HDL** (every lab visit)
- **Sleep** (nightly): hours, quality, and consistency (aim for 6-9 hours a night)
- **Energy** (daily): morning vs afternoon crash
- **Cravings** (daily): especially "I need sugar now" feelings
- **Feet check** (daily): sensation, sores, redness
- **Vision** (weekly): sudden blurriness, floaters, dark spots, changes

These are not random metrics. They are the places diabetes tries to collect interest.

A quick reality story

Let me paint two short scenes, based on common patterns seen in clinics (not specific individuals):

Jason, 66, thought diabetes was just "high sugar." He took multiple meds, kept "managing," and felt older every year. What finally scared him was not his A1C. It was numb toes and a blurry spot that came and went. Those symptoms made it real.

Becky, 62, carried years of severe insulin resistance. She was exhausted in a way sleep did not fix. Walking felt like dragging a heavy backpack. When her plan shifted toward reducing insulin overload with structured nutrition changes and carefully supervised medication adjustments, she did not just see better numbers. She felt her body come back online.

The point is not that everyone will get the same results. The point is that when you treat Type 2 like a whole-body problem, you stop playing defense.

Coming next

Now you understand why diabetes is not "just blood sugar."

So the next question is unavoidable:

What is driving insulin resistance in the first place?

In Step 2, we're going to name the real driver clearly: **hyperinsulinemia**, meaning chronically high insulin. You will learn why it happens, why it gets normalized, and why lowering insulin levels safely is one of the most powerful levers for reversing the Type 2 process.

STEP 2 - Understand the Real Issue: Hyperinsulinemia

Insulin First, Glucose Later

H ere's an uplifting fact to start with: in a major clinical trial, people at high risk cut their chances of developing type 2 diabetes by **58%** using lifestyle changes, without any new magic drug. That is not a tiny effect. That is a "your future can look different" effect. (New England Journal of Medicine)

Now let's talk about the trap most people fall into.

If you've ever felt like your body is betraying you, you are not crazy. You did the "right" things. You ate less. You counted. You tried to be good. And you still gained weight or your blood sugar still crept up. You might even have been told, directly or indirectly, that the problem is your discipline.

That blame is convenient. It is also incomplete.

The "diabesity" clue nobody explained

Type 2 diabetes and weight gain often show up together so often that researchers sometimes talk about them like one big problem: diabetes + obesity. The combo matters because it hints at a shared driver underneath.

Most people are taught to stare at **glucose** like it's the villain. Glucose is important, but it is often the smoke, not the fire.

The fire, for many people, is **too much insulin for too long**, also called **hyperinsulinemia**.

Calories are real, but the "calorie story" is missing the main character

Yes, energy matters. But the body is not a simple bank account where you deposit food calories and withdraw exercise calories.

Your body is more like a phone with an adaptive battery. When you keep trying to run it on low power, it quietly changes settings in the background. Research on calorie restriction shows energy expenditure can drop more than you would expect from weight loss alone, a phenomenon often called metabolic adaptation. (PubMed Central)

And here's the crucial point for this chapter: **hormones decide where energy goes.**

You can't "choose" to feel less hungry at 10 p.m. when you are stressed, sleep-deprived, and your brain wants quick comfort. Hunger and satiety are regulated. The system is not weak. It's powerful.

Insulin is one of the strongest signals in that system.

The hidden timeline: insulin often rises before glucose

This is the part that changes how you see type 2 diabetes.

In the years before a type 2 diagnosis, many people's bodies start to become less responsive to insulin. To keep blood glucose looking "normal," the pancreas compensates by making **more insulin**. That means **insulin can be high while glucose still looks fine**, especially on basic screening labs.

In the Whitehall II study, researchers tracked people for years and saw measurable shifts in insulin sensitivity and insulin secretion **years before** diabetes was diagnosed. Glucose rose sharply close to diagnosis, but the underlying insulin changes showed up earlier. (PubMed)

So if you only watch glucose, it can feel like diabetes "appears out of nowhere."

It usually doesn't. It builds.

Symptom vs driver: a simple mental model

Think of glucose as traffic on a highway.

- **Glucose** is the number of cars.
- **Insulin** is the traffic control system telling cars where to go, where to park, and when to stop.

If the traffic system is blasting "PARK EVERYTHING" all day, the parking lots fill. Then the shoulders fill. Then the side streets fill. Eventually, traffic backs up on the highway itself. That "backup" is the high blood sugar you can finally see.

Here's a "cause vs symptom" flow you can use:

Frequent high-insulin signals (food choices + constant eating + stress + poor sleep)

→ **more storage** (especially around organs)

→ **insulin resistance increases** (cells stop listening)

→ **insulin rises even more** (pancreas compensates)

→ **glucose rises** (compensation starts failing)

→ **type 2 diagnosis**

This is why **hyperinsulinemia can come first**. Glucose is often the late-stage alarm.

Why belly fat is such a loud warning sign

Not all body fat behaves the same. Fat stored deep in the abdomen, around organs (often called visceral fat), tracks more strongly with metabolic risk than "pinchable" fat under the skin.

Large studies show that waist-related measures can add useful information beyond BMI for predicting type 2 diabetes risk. (BMJ)

And waist-to-height ratio has been linked with mortality risk and "years of life lost," with a simple public message: keep your waist less than half your height. (PLOS)

Here's the uncomfortable but empowering truth: someone can look "not that overweight" and still have high-risk fat stored internally. That's one reason the scale can lie.

Why removing fat doesn't fix the problem

If fat were the main cause, then removing fat should fix the metabolism.

But in a well-known study, large-volume liposuction removed significant subcutaneous fat and did **not** meaningfully improve insulin sensitivity or major metabolic risk factors. (PubMed)

That does not mean fat is meaningless. It means fat is often a **storage outcome** of the deeper hormonal environment.

Step 2 actionables: what raises insulin in real life

You don't need perfection. You need awareness and a plan.

1) Food triggers that commonly spike insulin

- **Sugary drinks** (soda, sweet coffee drinks, energy drinks, many "juice" drinks)Sugar-sweetened beverages are consistently associated with higher type 2 diabetes risk in meta-analyses. (PubMed Central)
- **Refined carbs** (pastries, white bread, white pasta, white bread, many breakfast cereals, candy, chips)
- **Ultra-processed snack foods** designed to be easy to overeat
- **Liquid calories** because they bypass fullness signals fast

2) Frequency triggers: the "always eating" problem

Even if portions are not huge, **constant grazing** keeps insulin from fully coming down. If insulin is the storage signal, it's like pressing and holding a button all day. Your body never gets a real "off" moment.

Quick Story:

John is 55, and his days follow the same exhausting rhythm. He skips breakfast and lunch, running on regular soda to get him through long hours, then sits down to one large dinner at night. By then, his blood sugars are already high. They stay high. His A1c never seems to improve, no matter how much he worries about it. What John doesn't see is what's happening inside his body: his pancreas is being pushed nonstop. All day, the steady stream of sugar from soda forces it to release insulin again and again, without relief. Then the large evening meal demands a massive insulin response all at once. Over time, this constant overwork wears the pancreas down, making it harder to keep blood sugars in range. John isn't failing. His pancreas is exhausted, trying to keep up with a pattern that gives it no rest.

Start simple:

- Pick **meals over random snacks**
- Build a predictable pattern (breakfast, lunch, dinner, or two meals if that fits your life and you feel good)

You're not doing this to punish yourself. You're doing it to stop blasting the signal.

3) Sleep and stress triggers that act like gasoline

Sleep loss and stress don't just affect mood. They hit metabolism.

- In a controlled study, restricting sleep to 4 hours per night for several nights worsened glucose tolerance and altered hormones like cortisol. (

PubMed)

· Chronic stress is linked to impaired insulin signaling through multiple biological pathways. (PubMed Central)

Marcus is 45 and works third shift. He sleeps only four to five broken hours a day while carrying the weight of a high stress job that never truly lets his body rest. Every morning his blood sugars run high, and every appointment brings the same frustration. His A1c will not come down no matter how hard he tries. He takes his medications, watches what he eats, and pushes through exhaustion, yet his body stays locked in survival mode. Chronic stress, sleep deprivation, and a flipped circadian rhythm quietly fuel insulin resistance. Marcus feels like he is failing, but the truth is far more complicated. He is not careless or unmotivated. He is exhausted, overworked, and managing diabetes in a world that was not built for night shift lives.

Translation: if you are living on low sleep and high stress, your body can act "insulin resistant" even before the diet is perfect.

Try this "minimum effective dose" approach:

· Protect a consistent sleep window as often as you can
· Use a 2-minute downshift routine (slow breathing, short walk, shower, journaling) before late-night eating happens

Optional lab talk with a clinician: fasting insulin and HOMA-IR

Most routine checkups emphasize fasting glucose and A1C. Useful, but they may miss the early phase where **insulin is high but glucose still looks okay**.

You can ask a clinician about:

· **Fasting insulin**
· **HOMA-IR**, which is a calculation using fasting glucose and fasting insulin, often used in research and sometimes in clinical settings (PubMed)

This is not about self-diagnosing. It's about seeing the driver earlier, so you can steer sooner.

The point of this chapter

If you remember one thing, make it this:

High glucose is often the moment the problem becomes visible.

Hyperinsulinemia is often the moment the problem becomes unstoppable, unless you intervene.

And you can intervene.

In the next chapter, we're going to make insulin feel obvious instead of mysterious. You'll learn insulin's real job, why your body treats it like a "store this now" command, and the metaphor that will make the whole system click: the **overpacked suitcase**.

Insulin: Storage Hormone

Here's an uplifting fact to start: in detailed metabolic studies, **liver fat can drop fast after weight loss**, and that shift is tightly linked to better blood sugar control in many people with type 2 diabetes (Taylor et al., 2018). That means your body is not "broken." It is responsive. It listens when the signal changes.

Now let's talk about the signal almost nobody explains clearly.

If I wanted to help someone gain weight quickly, I would not hand them a bag of chips and say "good luck." I would do something far more direct.

I would raise their insulin.

That sounds dramatic, but it's not a conspiracy theory. In real life, **weight gain is a common side effect when insulin therapy is intensified**, especially in people with type 2 diabetes (Pontiroli et al., 2011; McFarlane et al., 2009). Doctors see it. Patients feel it. Pants confirm it.

This is not because insulin is "bad." Insulin is essential. Without it, you cannot use food properly. People with untreated type 1 diabetes lose weight rapidly because glucose cannot get into cells and the body goes into emergency breakdown mode.

Insulin is more like a powerful manager. When it shows up, it gives commands. The big command is simple:

Store energy. Save it. Pack it away.

And that brings us to the real job of insulin.

Insulin is not just a blood sugar hormone

Most people hear "insulin" and think "blood sugar." That is like hearing "coach" and thinking "whistle." The whistle matters, but the coach runs the whole game.

Insulin helps move nutrients into tissues and helps decide what the body does next with that energy. In plain language, insulin tends to do three things:

1. **Get fuel into cells**
2. **Turn extra fuel into stored energy**
3. **Block stored energy from being released**

That third one is the part that changes everything.

Insulin is one of the strongest "do not open the pantry" signals your body has.

In adipose tissue, insulin **suppresses lipolysis**, which is the breakdown of stored fat into fatty acids that can be used for energy (Santoro et al., 2021; Carpentier, 2021). In other words, insulin does not only help you store. It also tells your body to pause burning what you already stored.

So when insulin stays high all day, your body is basically hearing:

"Keep storing. Stop releasing. Stay in storage mode."

The body has two energy banks

Your body stores energy in two main forms:

1) Glycogen

This is stored glucose, packed into chains, mainly in the liver and muscles. It is fast-access energy. Like cash in your wallet.

2) Body fat (triglycerides)

This is long-term storage, mostly in fat cells. More like money in a savings account.

After you eat, insulin rises. That helps push glucose into cells and also helps refill glycogen. But glycogen storage is limited. When those "wallet" pockets fill up, the body starts putting more into savings.

That is where the liver gets involved.

The liver: your body's shipping warehouse

Think of your liver like a busy warehouse that sorts and ships nutrients.

When extra glucose keeps arriving, the liver does not just shrug. It adapts.

One pathway is called **de novo lipogenesis**, which means "making new fat." When carbohydrate intake is high and the hormonal environment favors storage, the liver can convert some of that excess into fat (Kersten, 2001; Sanders & Griffin, 2016). This process is studied heavily in fatty liver disease and insulin resistance, because it is one way fat builds up where you do not want it, including inside the liver (Smith et al., 2020).

Then the liver packages triglycerides for transport, often in particles called **VLDL**, and sends them out into the bloodstream. Over time, those triglycerides can be delivered to fat tissue for storage (Zammit, 2001).

None of this happens because your body hates you. It happens because your body is trying to protect you from having too much glucose floating around.

Glucose is useful, but too much of it in the wrong place is damaging. So the body stores it. Insulin is the "store it" message.

Storage mode vs burn mode

Here is a simple mental model you can replay any time you are confused:

When insulin is high, you are mostly in storage mode.

When insulin is low, you can access burn mode.

Burn mode is when your body can tap glycogen and fat to power your day.

This is why constant eating is such a problem, even when calories look "reasonable." If insulin rarely drops, burn mode rarely turns on.

You can work out, count calories, and still feel like you are pushing a boulder uphill if your body is hearing "store" all day.

The "overpacked suitcase" metaphor

Now let's use the signature metaphor that will carry the next chapters.
Imagine your body has a suitcase for energy.

- Glycogen is the easy-to-reach items on top.
- Fat storage is everything packed deeper inside.

Insulin is the person trying to zip the suitcase closed.

When you eat frequently, insulin keeps pressing down, trying to make everything fit. At first, it works. The suitcase closes.

But if you keep stuffing snacks, sugary drinks, and "little bites" all day, the suitcase gets **overpacked**.

Now the zipper strains. The seams stretch. You sit on it to force it shut.

That "sitting on the suitcase" is what high insulin does in the body: it forces storage even when storage capacity is getting overwhelmed.

And when the suitcase is overpacked, a new problem appears:

Your cells start resisting insulin's push.

Not because you failed. Not because you are lazy. Because the suitcase is full.

That is insulin resistance, which is the next chapter. But before we go there, you need one more key truth.

Why insulin can make weight gain easier

If insulin makes it easier to store energy and harder to release stored energy, then two people can eat similar calories and have different outcomes depending on the hormonal environment.

This is why weight gain often shows up when insulin therapy is intensified (Pontiroli et al., 2011), and why medications that increase insulin secretion, such as sulfonylureas, are commonly associated with weight gain compared to metformin in research comparing treatments (Hemmingsen et al., 2014).

On the flip side, metformin lowers glucose mostly by reducing liver glucose output and improving insulin sensitivity, and it is often weight neutral or modestly weight reducing (Yerevanian & Shulman, 2019; Haber et al., 2024).

You do not need to memorize drug names. You only need the pattern:

- **More insulin signaling tends to push storage and weight gain.**
- **Less insulin signaling makes it easier to access stored fuel.**

Again, insulin is not evil. Insulin is powerful.

What actually keeps insulin high all day

Some triggers are obvious, like sugary drinks and refined carbs.

But the sneaky trigger is frequency.

A lot of people live in a pattern like this:

- quick breakfast
- mid-morning snack
- sweet coffee drink
- lunch
- "just one" treat
- afternoon snack
- dinner
- night snack while scrolling

None of those moments feels huge. But together, they create a day where insulin rarely gets a real break.

And if insulin never gets a break, fat burning feels locked behind a door.

Actionables: stop the constant signal

You are not trying to "eat perfectly." You are trying to stop sending the storage message every two hours.

Here are practical moves that work in real life. Getting back to basics with a planned eating pattern can help.

1) Build meal structure you can actually keep

Pick a structure that fits your schedule and your hunger. Examples:

- **3 meals, no snacks**
- **3 meals, one planned snack**
- **2 meals, one planned snack** (some people feel great here)

The magic is not the number. The magic is that it is planned. Consistent carbohydrate intake at set times throughout the day can actually help to balance blood sugars.

Planned beats random.

If you already take glucose-lowering meds, especially insulin or sulfony-lureas, do not change meal timing drastically without a clinician's guidance because hypoglycemia risk is real.

2) Make meals "stick" so you do not hunt for food an hour later

A meal that holds you usually has:

- a solid protein source
- fiber-rich plants
- enough fat to slow digestion
- a carb choice that is not pure sugar

Teen-friendly examples:

- Eggs plus Greek yogurt plus berries
- Chicken bowl with beans, veggies, salsa, and avocado
- Tuna or tofu wrap with crunchy vegetables and olive-oil-based dressing
- Chili with extra vegetables and a side salad

This is not "diet food." This is "I want my brain to stop screaming for snacks" food.

3) Shrink snacking without feeling punished

If snacking is currently your comfort, your reward, your stress shield, or your "I'm bored" button, ripping it away overnight can backfire.

Try a step-down approach:

- Week 1: Replace one snack with a higher-protein option.
- Week 2: Make snacks planned and consistent.
- Week 3: Test a snack-free gap between lunch and dinner.

Better snack options if you truly need one:

- nuts plus fruit
- cheese or yogurt
- jerky and an apple
- carrots and hummus

These tend to create a smaller insulin rollercoaster than candy, pastries, or sweet drinks.

4) Kill the liquid sugar habit first

This is the fastest win for many people because it is so common and so easy to underestimate.

If you drink your calories, your body often does not register fullness the same way it does with chewing.

Swap ideas:

- soda to sparkling water
- sweet latte to unsweetened coffee with milk
- juice to whole fruit
- energy drink to water plus a walk plus real sleep when possible

5) Give insulin a "down time" window

You do not need heroic fasting. You need consistency.

A simple target many people can tolerate:

- finish dinner
- no calories for a few hours before bed
- no late-night snack unless truly needed

Late-night eating is often not hunger. It is stress, habit, and dopamine. If that is you, you are not weak. You are human. Skipping meals through the day can also cause us to overeat at night. Something that works for me is distracting myself when I get the urge to open the fridge. Distractions can be something like a short walk when I have the urge to go to the fridge, petting my cat or opening my notebook and writing my thoughts and worries.

Try a replacement ritual:

- brush teeth early
- drink herbal tea
- put a sticky note on your snack cabinet: "Am I hungry or tired?"
- do a 2-minute stretch or shower

Tiny rituals beat willpower battles.

The point of this chapter

Insulin is the master storage hormone.

When insulin rises, your body stores energy. When insulin stays high too often, your body stores more, releases less, and eventually struggles to respond to insulin normally.

That is not a moral failure. It is biology.

And it sets up the most important question of the whole reset:

What happens when the suitcase is overpacked and the zipper stops moving?

That is the next chapter, where we turn insulin resistance into an "overflow" story you can finally understand, and stop blaming yourself for a system that has been pushed past capacity.

A Quick Blessing

Your feedback is a true blessing!

If this book has encouraged you, helped you feel hopeful or gave you some useful tools, would you leave a quick review?

Even one sentence makes a huge difference and takes just a minute. As a small author, your feedback not only lifts my heart... It also helps others find the support and hope they need.

Thank you for being part of this journey!

Scan this QR code with your phone to go to the review page

Or

Go to your orders, find the book and click

"Write a product review"

Thank you <3

STEP 3 — See Insulin Resistance as "Overflow"

STEP 3 — See Insulin Resistance as "Overflow"

The Overflow Phenomenon

Uplifting fact: Your cells can become *more* insulin-sensitive in days when you stop flooding them with constant fuel, because insulin resistance is not a life sentence. It is often a *reversible traffic jam.* (BMJ)

Picture this. You are doing "everything right." You cut back. You walk more. You white-knuckle your cravings. And still your blood sugar stays stubborn. Still your belly feels like it has its own gravity. Still you wake up tired, like your sleep did not fully load.

That feeling is terrifying because it comes with a quiet fear: *What if my body is broken?*

Here is the twist: most of the time, your body is not broken. It is protecting you.

Insulin resistance is not laziness

Insulin resistance sounds like your body is being stubborn on purpose, like a teenager ignoring a text. But biologically, it is more like a smoke alarm that will not stop beeping because the kitchen is already full of smoke.

Resistance is one of the body's oldest survival skills. When something stays high for too long, your body pushes back to keep you alive. That is homeostasis: the internal "autopilot" that fights extreme swings. (Diabetes Journals)

We see this everywhere:

- Loud noise becomes background noise.
- Drugs lose their "hit" over time.
- Germs become resistant when exposed constantly.

The pattern is simple: **exposure creates resistance.**

Now apply that to insulin.

When insulin stays high too often, for too long, your body protects itself by responding less to it. In other words: **high, persistent insulin can *cause* insulin resistance.** (PubMed Central)

That is not a motivational quote. Scientists have literally induced insulin resistance by keeping insulin elevated for days. In one classic study, healthy people given chronic insulin infusion developed a significant drop in insulin-mediated glucose disposal, roughly **20 to 40%** in about **72 hours**. (Springer Link)

So insulin resistance is not just "bad luck." It is often the body saying:

"I cannot keep shoving more energy into cells that are already full."

The overflow model: why insulin "can't do its job"

The old story goes like this: insulin is a key, your cell is a lock, and in insulin resistance the lock is broken.

But there's a problem. In type 2 diabetes, the insulin "key" and the receptor "lock" are usually structurally normal. The bigger issue is what happens *inside*

47

the cell, especially in the liver. (PubMed Central)

Here is the overflow model, in plain language:

- **Your liver and muscle cells are like suitcases.**
- Insulin is the person trying to zip the suitcase shut.
- Sugar and stored fuel are the clothes.

If the suitcase is half-empty, insulin can zip it easily and store energy safely.

But if the suitcase is already stuffed, the zipper fights back. You can yank harder, but it just gets worse. That yanking is what we do when we respond to insulin resistance by pushing insulin higher and higher, either by the body producing more or by giving larger doses. (Springer Link)

Overflow visual you can imagine right now: the full sink.

- The sink is your cell.
- The water is incoming fuel (glucose, fructose, stored energy).
- The drain is your ability to burn fuel between meals.

If the faucet is on all day (constant eating, frequent snacking, sugary drinks), the sink eventually fills. When it is full, water spills over onto the counter. That spillover is high blood sugar.

Now, what does "try harder" do? It often turns the faucet down a tiny bit, but keeps it running all day.

The real win is turning the faucet off long enough for the drain to catch up.

Why "try harder" is not the fix

Most people attack insulin resistance with a brutal strategy: more willpower.

- White-knuckle portion control.
- Fight hunger all day.
- Exercise like you are paying off a debt.

The problem is that willpower is not a hormone. Insulin is.

When insulin stays elevated, your body is being instructed to store and protect stored energy. That can make fat loss feel like pushing a car uphill in the rain. (PubMed Central)

Also, your body adapts. If you constantly force a deficit with constant hunger, your brain starts negotiating: cravings rise, energy drops, and your focus gets shaky. (We will go deeper on that in Chapter 8.)

So instead of "try harder," you need a better lever:

Lower the overflow.

The "drain the overflow" plan

You are not trying to "beat" your body. You are trying to give it room to breathe.

Here are the practical moves that drain the sink and unzip the suitcase.

1) Create insulin breaks every day

Insulin should rise and fall. That up-and-down rhythm helps prevent resistance. (PubMed Central)

Try this progression:

- **Week 1:** Stop eating after dinner. Aim for a **12-hour overnight break** (example: 8 pm to 8 am).
- **Week 2:** Add an extra hour, **13 hours**.
- **Week 3:** Try **14 hours** most days if it feels okay.

This is not punishment. It is giving your body time to use what is already stored.

Safety note: If you use insulin or sulfonylureas, fasting can cause low blood sugar. Do not adjust medications alone. Get clinical guidance. (Diabetes Journals)

2) Remove "liquid overflow"

If you do only one thing, do this.

Soda, sweet coffee drinks, juice, energy drinks: they pour fuel in fast, with almost no chewing, no fullness, and a big insulin response. It is like dumping buckets into an already-full sink.

Swap to:

- Water (sparkling is fine)
- Unsweetened tea
- Black coffee or coffee with minimal added sugar

3) Build meals that do not spike the faucet

A simple template:

- **Protein first** (eggs, Greek yogurt, chicken, tofu, fish)
- **Fiber next** (vegetables, beans, lentils, berries)
- **Smart carbs last** (whole foods, not refined)
- **Add healthy fat** for steadier energy (olive oil, nuts, avocado)

You are not "dieting." You are reducing how fast fuel rushes in.

4) Move after meals to "open storage space"

A 10-15 minute walk after eating can help pull glucose into muscles without demanding huge insulin. Think of it as making extra room in the suitcase. (PubMed Central)

It does not need to be intense. Consistency beats drama.

5) Sleep like it matters (because it does)

Sleep loss can worsen insulin sensitivity and crank up hunger. If your sleep is chaotic, your body behaves like it is under threat, and it stores fuel like winter is coming. (PubMed Central)

Aim for a boring, repeatable bedtime.

A quick story to make this real

Philip was 46 and dealing with a diabetic foot ulcer that would not heal. Ten months. Dressings. Specialist visits. Antibiotics. The kind of problem that can end in amputation.

He started a simple rhythm: a structured fasting practice once a week, and a calmer eating pattern the rest of the time. Within a month, his blood sugar readings normalized enough that he stopped his diabetes meds with medical supervision. His ulcer healed. Over the year, he lost weight and kept his A1C lower than when he was on multiple medications.

The point is not that fasting is magic. The point is that **when the overflow drops, your body stops fighting you.**

Teaser for next chapter

Now that you see insulin resistance as overflow, something shocking becomes obvious:

Weight loss is not the strategy. It is the *receipt*.

The strategy is lowering the overflow that forced your body to store.

That is exactly what we are tackling next.

Weight Follows Health

Uplifting fact: In a major clinical trial, many people with type 2 diabetes achieved remission through a structured approach that reduced internal fat and improved metabolism, and success was strongly tied to reducing the underlying "fuel overload." (The Lancet)

Let's be honest: weight loss advice can feel like an endless lecture.

"Eat less."

"Move more."

"Be disciplined."

And if you struggle, the world acts like it is a character flaw.

But if you understand overflow, you can finally stop blaming yourself for biology.

Why weight loss helps (and why it's not the first move)

Weight loss often improves blood sugar because it usually means less fat stored in the wrong places, especially **visceral fat** and **fat inside the liver**. When liver fat drops, the liver can respond to insulin better and stops leaking extra glucose into the blood. (PubMed Central)

That is why weight loss helps.

But here's the trap: **chasing weight loss directly** often backfires because it keeps you focused on the scoreboard instead of the game.

The real target is the hidden overflow:

- high fasting insulin
- fatty liver
- visceral fat
- constant snacking cycles

When you lower those, weight tends to follow.

"Obesity is hormonal" (said carefully and accurately)

Calories matter. They are real energy.

But hormones decide what your body does with that energy: store it, burn it, or scream for more food.

Insulin is one of the strongest storage signals we have. When insulin is high often, fat storage becomes easier and fat burning becomes harder. That does not mean insulin is the only hormone involved, but it is a major one in this story. (PubMed Central)

This also explains something that confuses people:

- Some people can be heavier and not develop type 2 diabetes.
- Some people can look "normal weight" and still have insulin resistance.

Because the issue is not only total body weight. It is *where the overflow is stored.*

Why focusing only on calories often fails in real life

Counting calories sounds clean on paper. In real life, it crashes into three messy realities:

1. **Hunger is not a moral issue.**If your food choices keep insulin high and blood sugar swinging, your appetite will feel louder. You can ignore it for a week. You cannot ignore it forever.
2. **Ultra-processed foods hijack your "off switch."**A handful of chips can turn into a whole bag before your brain even registers fullness.
3. **The scale is a liar sometimes.**Salt, stress, sleep, hormones, and inflammation can move scale weight quickly even when you are improving internally.

If your only win condition is "scale down," you will quit on weeks when your body is actually healing.

53

Measure what matters: waist over scale

If overflow is the issue, your best at-home signal is often your **waist circumference**, because it tracks abdominal fat better than weight alone. Major medical groups have argued waist should be used routinely because it can improve cardiometabolic risk assessment beyond BMI. (PubMed Central)

How to measure your waist (simple, repeatable):

- Stand relaxed.
- Measure around your abdomen (commonly at the level of the belly button, using the same spot each time).
- Do it once weekly, same time of day, same conditions.

Also useful: **waist-to-height ratio** (waist less than half your height is a common rule of thumb used in research discussions of risk screening). (PubMed)

When the waist shrinks, overflow is draining.

Actionables: make health the strategy

Here is your "weight follows health" checklist. These are not slogans. These are levers.

1) Pick 2 insulin-lowering habits and lock them in

Examples:

- 12–14 hour overnight eating break
- No liquid sugar
- Protein-first breakfast
- 10-minute walk after dinner

Win with consistency, not perfection.

2) Strength training: the "extra closet space" move

Muscle is a place to store glucose safely. More muscle can mean more room for fuel, less overflow pressure. Keep it simple:

- 2–3 sessions/week
- Push, pull, squat/hinge basics
- Start light, progress slowly

3) Stop "all-or-nothing" eating

When you think you "blew it," you tend to turn one imperfect meal into a weekend.

Instead, use this rule: **Next meal normal.**

That single habit keeps insulin spikes from turning into a full overflow relapse.

4) Watch for the quiet wins

If these improve, you are moving in the right direction:

- less afternoon crash
- fewer cravings at night
- waking up less puffy
- smaller waist
- steadier mood

Those are metabolic victories.

Callout to remember

"You don't lose weight to get healthy. You get healthy and weight follows."

Teaser for the next chapter

Now we need to talk about the biggest lie people are told when they try to fix this:

"Just eat less."

What happens when you chronically restrict, get hungrier, slow down, and then blame yourself for quitting?

In the next chapter, we expose **The Calorie Deception** and why "eat less" can backfire, even when you are trying your hardest.

The Calorie Trap

Uplifting fact: In controlled studies, people with type 2 diabetes often improve blood sugar in as little as **weeks** when they change the *kind* of food and the *timing* of meals, even before dramatic weight loss shows up. (BMJ)

If you have ever tried to "just eat less," you already know the dirty secret: it can feel like your body is fighting you. You cut portions, you track every bite, you go to bed hungry, and the scale might barely move. Then one stressful week hits, you eat normally again, and it feels like your body snaps back fast.

That is not you being weak. That is biology being stubborn.

This chapter is about the **calorie deception**: the idea that your body is a simple math problem. Calories in, calories out, done. That sounds logical until you realize your body is not a calculator. It is more like a phone with an aggressive "battery saver mode." When fuel drops, your body quietly turns down background systems to survive.

And if you are living with insulin resistance, the calorie trap gets even nastier, because the problem is not only how much energy you eat. It is **where that**

energy gets stored and whether your cells are already full.

Why low-calorie plans often backfire

Let's make this visual.

Picture a campfire. You want it to burn bright. You remove half the wood (calorie restriction). The fire does not politely keep burning at the same rate. It slows down. Your body does that too.

Researchers call this **adaptive thermogenesis**, basically your metabolism adjusting downward after weight loss or calorie restriction, making weight regain more likely. (PubMed) In real people, long-term studies have found that resting energy use can stay lower than expected even years after major weight loss. (PubMed Central)

So when someone says, "Just eat 500 calories less per day," they are assuming your "calories out" stays stable. But your body can respond by:

- burning fewer calories at rest
- making you feel colder and more tired
- making you think about food constantly

None of that is a character flaw. It is a survival feature.

The low-fat, low-calorie era: a reality check

For decades, official advice pushed a low-fat pattern that often meant higher carbs. The pitch was simple: lower fat, lower calories, better heart health, easier weight loss.

Then large, expensive trials tested versions of that idea in the real world.

In the **Women's Health Initiative Dietary Modification Trial**, tens of thousands of women were assigned to a low-fat dietary pattern for years. The results did not match the hype. Weight changes were modest, and cardiovascular outcomes did not dramatically improve the way people expected. (PubMed)

In **Look AHEAD,** more than 5,000 adults with type 2 diabetes were assigned to an intensive lifestyle program aiming for weight loss and improved fitness. After a median follow-up of **9.6 years**, the main cardiovascular outcome did not improve enough, and the intervention was stopped early for futility. (New England Journal of Medicine)

This does not mean lifestyle is pointless. It means one specific strategy, "eat less, move more, low-fat it," often fails to deliver the promised big wins.

The teen and young adult problem: "Even when they try, it still gets worse"

Now the scary part.

In the **TODAY** trial (Treatment Options for Type 2 Diabetes in Adolescents and Youth), researchers tested treatments in youth with type 2 diabetes, including a lifestyle intervention added to metformin. Over time, a large portion still lost glycemic control. The lifestyle add-on did not magically fix the disease. (New England Journal of Medicine)

If motivated young people, with structured support, struggle to control type 2 diabetes with the classic model, it tells us something important:

Willpower is not the main lever. Biology is.

Hunger hormones: why "eat less" feels like torture

Here is what calorie math ignores: your hunger is not a motivational quote. It is a **hormone-driven alarm system.**

- **Ghrelin** tends to rise and push hunger.
- **PYY** and **CCK** tend to signal fullness.
- Other signals, including gut-brain hormones, influence cravings, reward, and appetite control.

This system evolved to keep you alive, not to keep you lean for selfies. (Royal Society Publishing)

So when you chronically restrict calories, your body often responds with stronger hunger signals and louder food thoughts. That is why "I'll just be disciplined forever" is a plan that collapses the moment life gets messy.

Exercise is powerful, but not the main weight-loss lever

Exercise is still one of the best things you can do for insulin resistance. It helps muscles pull glucose from the blood, improves fitness, helps mood, and can lower A1C. Structured training is linked to meaningful A1C reductions in type 2 diabetes. (JAMA Network)

But exercise alone often disappoints for fat loss because humans compensate. Some people get hungrier, some move less the rest of the day, and some "reward eat" without noticing. A systematic review found that reductions in non-exercise activity can happen during diet or exercise interventions, which helps explain "less-than-expected" weight loss. (Cambridge University Press & Assessment)

So the truth is nuanced:

· **Exercise is medicine for metabolism.**
· **Food timing and food type are usually the bigger levers for fat loss and blood sugar.**

The real issue: not energy excess, energy traffic

This is the shift that changes everything.

If your body is insulin resistant, the problem is not only "too many calories."

It is **too much energy being pushed into storage**, especially into places it does not belong.

Think of insulin like a **traffic cop** directing fuel.

· When insulin is high, your body tends to store more and burn less.
· When insulin is lower, your body can access stored fuel more easily.

That is why two diets with the same calories can feel totally different in your body. One can leave you starving and tired. The other can feel calm, steady, and doable.

And this is why the new strategy is not "eat less."

It is:

Eat differently, and sometimes eat intermittently.

Actionables: build a deficit without misery

Use these as a practical reset. You are not chasing perfection. You are building an environment where your body stops screaming for snacks.

1) "Eat differently" checklist

Aim for meals that are **low in refined carbs** and **high in protein and fiber**, with healthy fats.

- Build each meal around: **protein + plants**
- examples: eggs and veggies, Greek yogurt and berries, chicken and salad, tofu stir-fry, tuna and crunchy vegetables
- Swap ultra-processed carbs for slower carbs
- replace soda and juice with water or zero-sugar drinks
- replace pastries and chips with fruit, nuts, cheese, or hummus
- Keep "liquid sugar" near zero most days
- it spikes blood sugar fast and does not fill you up

Low and very low carbohydrate approaches, on average, improve A1C and can increase rates of diabetes remission at least in the shorter term for some people. (BMJ)

2) "Eat intermittently" starter plan

Do not start with heroic fasts. Start with a pattern your life can handle.

- **Step 1:** 12-hour overnight break (example: finish dinner at 8 pm, first meal at 8 am)
- **Step 2:** 14 hours on 3 to 5 days per week
- **Step 3:** If you tolerate it, try 16 hours occasionally

Your goal is not punishment. Your goal is to reduce constant insulin "background noise" from nonstop snacking. If fasting causes you to eat more later in the day than go back to a normal eating pattern of three meals a day.

3) Use the "after-meal walk" hack

A 10 to 15 minute easy walk after meals is a cheat code because it helps muscles soak up glucose. Keep it simple and consistent. (No special gear, no gym anxiety.)

4) Strength training twice per week

Even basic bodyweight moves count: squats to a chair, wall push-ups, bands, light dumbbells. More muscle means more storage space for glucose, which helps blood sugar stability over time. (JAMA Network)

5) Measure what matters

Do not let the scale bully you. Track **waist circumference** weekly. When insulin resistance improves, the waist often changes before the mirror mood does.

Safety note

If you use insulin or medications that can cause low blood sugar (like sulfonylureas), fasting or rapid carb reduction can trigger hypoglycemia. Make changes with medical guidance and monitor glucose. (Diabetes Journals)

What to remember

The calorie model is not totally wrong. It is just incomplete.

Your body is not a passive bucket. It is a regulated system with hormones, brakes, and alarms. If you try to force fat loss by raw restriction, your body often fights back with lower energy use and louder hunger.

The better play is to **lower the signal that drives storage**, create space in the system, and let weight loss become a side effect.

Next, we get even more specific: **why the real bottleneck is often inside the organs**, especially the liver, and how clearing that traffic jam changes everything.

STEP 4 — Fix the Organ Bottleneck: Fatty Liver + Visceral Fat

Chapter 9 — Fatty Liver Comes First

Uplifting fact: liver fat can drop fast. In controlled studies, reducing carbs can lower liver fat in just days, even before huge scale weight loss shows up. Your body responds quicker than your mirror does. (OUP Academic)

Now the hook you probably need to hear, even if it stings:

Most people do not wake up one day with type 2 diabetes. They walk into it, quietly, for years, while their liver is doing overtime in the dark.

That is why fatty liver is such a big deal. It is not just "a liver problem." It is a **traffic jam problem** that slows down your whole metabolism and makes blood sugar harder and harder to control. (The Lancet)

The silent step before diabetes

Fatty liver used to be called NAFLD (non-alcoholic fatty liver disease). Many medical groups now use **MASLD** (metabolic dysfunction-associated steatotic liver disease) because it highlights the real driver: metabolic dysfunction, especially insulin resistance. (aasld.org)

Here is the scary part: fatty liver is often silent. No pain. No obvious symptoms. Sometimes your liver enzymes are "normal" on a blood test, and you still have too much fat inside the liver. (Mayo Clinic)

And here is the motivating part:

Fatty liver is also one of the earliest warning lights that your blood sugar system is under strain. People with fatty liver are more likely to develop type 2 diabetes later. Even people who are not "obese" can have fatty liver and higher diabetes risk. (ScienceDirect)

So if you have ever thought, "My numbers are only a little high, I'm probably fine," this chapter is your friendly reality check.

Your liver is the body's traffic controller

Every time you eat, your bloodstream becomes a highway filled with:

- glucose (sugar energy)
- amino acids (protein building blocks)
- fats (fuel and storage)

Your liver sits like a traffic controller at a busy airport. It decides what gets stored, what gets burned, and what gets shipped out.

When the liver is lean and calm, it does three useful things:

1. Stores some glucose as glycogen (quick energy battery).
2. Releases glucose between meals to keep you stable.
3. Packages and ships fats in a controlled way.

When the liver is stuffed with fat, it becomes a stressed-out controller in a thunderstorm. Planes stack up. Delays spread.

That is what "fatty liver comes first" means.

How fatty liver pushes blood sugar up

Fatty liver and blood sugar are linked through a simple chain:

1. **Too much incoming sugar (especially refined carbs and fructose)** tells insulin to rise.
2. The liver stores glycogen until it is full.
3. Extra sugar gets converted into fat through **de novo lipogenesis (DNL)**, which literally means "making new fat." (PubMed Central)
4. Fat builds up inside the liver.
5. A fat-filled liver becomes **insulin resistant**, meaning insulin knocks but the liver does not listen well. (Nature)
6. The liver keeps releasing glucose even when you do not need it, especially overnight.
7. Your fasting blood sugar creeps up. Your A1C follows.

So the liver is not "lazy." It is **overloaded**.

The "saturated fat in blood" trap, explained carefully

This is where people get confused, so let's make it crystal clear.

Saturated fat in your blood is not always the same thing as saturated fat in your diet.

Your blood fats reflect your *metabolic state*.

When you eat lots of refined carbs and sugar, your liver can turn that sugar into fat through DNL. The fats created by DNL tend to be more saturated, like palmitate. (Springer Link)

That means someone can have higher "circulating saturated fats" even if they are not eating butter all day. In some studies, increasing dietary carbohydrate promotes blood markers linked to DNL, and dietary saturated fat and blood saturated fat are not always tightly matched. (PLOS)

Important nuance (no drama, just truth):

- Overeating calories from almost any source can increase liver fat.
- Some overfeeding studies suggest saturated fat can be especially harmful to the liver compared with unsaturated fat in that context. (ora.ox.ac.uk)

So the point is not "fat is good" or "fat is bad."

The point is: **a sugar-loaded, insulin-high state makes the liver manufacture and store fat.** And that fat changes how your liver handles glucose.

Why triglycerides and fatty liver travel together

When your liver makes extra fat, it tries to ship it out in particles called VLDL. That raises blood triglycerides. High-carb diets and alcohol consumption can increase triglycerides quickly in many people. (PubMed)

This matters because a common pattern shows up long before type 2 diabetes is diagnosed:

- rising waistline
- rising triglycerides
- falling HDL (the "good" cholesterol)
- slightly rising fasting glucose

That cluster is the metabolic syndrome vibe. It is your body whispering, then shouting: "Too much sugar traffic. Too much liver pressure." (The Lancet)

The most important mindset shift in Step 4

You are not fighting your body.

You are removing a bottleneck.

When the liver bottleneck clears, glucose control often improves because the whole system can breathe again.

And yes, this can happen even before you lose a ton of weight. That is part of why this chapter matters.

Actionables: 3 liver-supporting levers

These are the levers that directly reduce liver traffic.

1) Remove the fructose load

Fructose is processed mainly in the liver, and high intake is strongly linked with liver fat and DNL. (PubMed Central)
  Do this for 14 days:

- No soda, juice, sweet tea, energy drinks, "sports drinks."
- No "healthy" sugar bombs: smoothies, bottled fruit juices, sweetened coffees.
- Treat dried fruit like candy. It is easy to overdo.
- Read labels for: sucrose, HFCS, fruit concentrate, "nectar."

Swap list (easy wins):

- Water + lemon or mint
- Sparkling water
- Unsweetened tea
- Coffee with cinnamon or a splash of milk

2) Reduce refined carbs (the liver's fastest clogger)

Refined carbs are like dumping sand into your engine. They spike glucose and insulin quickly, feeding the liver overflow.
  Your refined-carb red flags:

- white bread, white bread, white pasta, white rice, bagels, pastries
- chips, crackers
- candy, cookies
- most boxed cereal

· "fat-free" snacks (often sugar-heavy)

Upgrade rule (simple):

If it came in a crinkly bag and disappears in your mouth in 30 seconds, it probably is not helping your liver.

Choose:

- whole foods
- more protein at meals
- high-fiber carbs if you eat them (beans, lentils, intact grains)
- vegetables as volume

3) Time-restrict your intake (so the liver has a night shift to clean up)

Time-restricted eating (TRE) means you eat within a consistent window, like 10 hours, and stop earlier at night. Trials and reviews suggest it can improve liver markers and liver fat in MASLD, though researchers still debate the "best" protocol. (PubMed Central)

Beginner TRE plan:

- Pick a 10-hour window.
- Example: 10:00 to 20:00.
- Water is always allowed.
- Try to stop eating 2 to 3 hours before sleep.

Why it helps:

Your liver gets a break from constant incoming fuel and can lower liver fat and improve insulin sensitivity over time. (PubMed Central)

Safety note (seriously):

If you take insulin or meds that can cause low blood sugar, do not change meal timing or fasting patterns without medical guidance. Hypoglycemia is real. (This book is "doctor-free" in spirit, not "ignore safety" in practice.)

Callout: Fructose and fatty liver resource

If you want a simple breakdown of fructose sources (including the "healthy" ones that sneak in), use the companion resource **"Fructose and Fatty Liver: The 10 Biggest Traps"** in the resources section of this book. (It is your label-reading cheat sheet.) (MDPI)

Visual: Liver as traffic controller (diagram)

FOOD IN
(refined carbs + fructose)

"Traffic Control"

Glycogen
(limited)

Fat
(DNL Overflow)

Glucose Output
(rises with resistance)

When DNL overflow rises:

✓ **Liver fat rises**

✓ **Insulin** resistance rises

✓ **Fasting glucose rises**

✓ **Triglycerides rise** (via VLDL export)

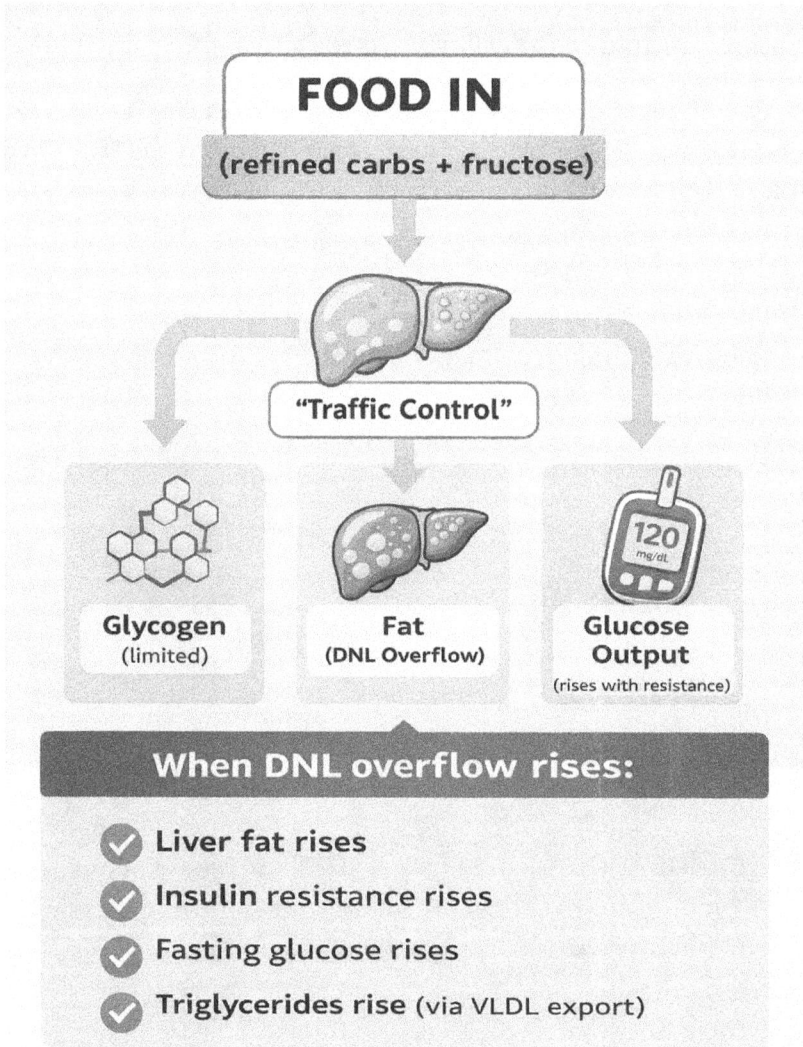

Keep this image in your head when you make food decisions. You are not "being good." You are clearing traffic.

Quick self-check: are you at risk for fatty liver?

This is not a diagnosis. It is a "pay attention" list.

- waist size increasing over months
- triglycerides trending up
- A1C or fasting glucose trending up
- blood pressure creeping up
- family history of type 2 diabetes
- constant snacking or late-night eating

Fatty liver is common in people with type 2 diabetes and metabolic syndrome, and it is tightly tied to cardiovascular risk too. (PubMed Central)

Closing: the calm liver advantage

When your liver stops being a storage closet for extra sugar, it becomes what it was designed to be: a smooth manager of energy.

That is the real "reset."

In the next chapter, we are going to get even more specific, because there is a brutal truth that changes everything:

Where fat is stored matters more than how much you have.

And once you learn how to measure that risk with nothing but a tape measure, you will never look at "weight" the same way again.

Chapter 10 — Fat Location Beats Fat Amount

Uplifting fact: shrinking your waist, even a little, can lower risk fast because visceral fat is one of the most "changeable" risk tissues when you remove sugar pressure, improve meals, and stop constant snacking. Waist is not just a number. It is a signal you can influence. (AHA Journals)

Let's start with a thought experiment.

Two people weigh the same.

Same height. Same BMI. Same "overweight" label.

Person A carries more fat under the skin, like a soft jacket.

Person B carries more fat deep in the belly, packed around organs.

Person B is usually in more danger, even if the scale is identical.

That is not fat-shaming. That is biology.

Visceral fat: the risky roommate

There are two main fat neighborhoods:

1. **Subcutaneous fat**The fat under your skin. You can pinch it.
2. **Visceral fat**The fat inside your abdomen, wrapped around organs like the liver, pancreas, and intestines.

Visceral fat is more strongly linked with insulin resistance, abnormal blood fats, and cardiometabolic risk than subcutaneous fat. (AHA Journals)

Why? Because visceral fat is not just stored energy. It acts more like an active, hormonal tissue that can flood the liver with fatty acids and inflammatory signals.

And remember Step 4: when the liver is overloaded, blood sugar control gets worse.

So yes, **your waistline can be more predictive than your weight.**

The simplest proxy for visceral fat: waist circumference

In a perfect world, everyone would get fancy body scans to measure visceral fat. In the real world, you have a tape measure.

Waist circumference is used in metabolic syndrome definitions and risk screening because it tracks central fat. (AHA Journals)

It is not perfect, but it is practical, cheap, and shockingly informative.

And here is the key: you are going to measure it correctly.

Actionable: the waist measurement protocol

Do this exactly the same way each time. Consistency beats perfection.

What you need

- Soft tape measure
- Notes app or a simple tracker
- 2 minutes

When to measure

- Morning, after using the bathroom
- Before eating or drinking
- Once per week (daily can mess with your head)

Where to measure (IDF method)

- Place the tape in a horizontal plane
- Midway between the lower rib margin and the top of the hip bone (iliac crest) (International Diabetes Federation)

How to measure

1. Stand tall, feet about hip-width.
2. Relax your belly. Do not "suck in." Do not push out.
3. Wrap the tape around, level all the way around (use a mirror).
4. Breathe out normally.
5. Read the number. Write it down.

Pro tip: take 2 readings. If they differ, take a third and use the middle one.

Tracking chart (copy and use)

Use centimeters or inches, but do not mix them.
You are not tracking to judge yourself.
You are tracking to see if your **organ bottleneck** is loosening.

The waist-risk ladder (simple version)

Risk thresholds vary by ethnicity and guidelines, but here is a useful ladder that shows the idea:

- **Higher risk begins around**Men: **94 cm** (about 37 in)Women: **80 cm** (about 31.5 in) (AHA Journals)
- **Risk is substantially higher around**Men: **102 cm** (about 40 in)Women: **88 cm** (about 35 in) (AHA Journals)

Again, this is a screening tool, not a life sentence.
Your mission is not "hit a perfect number."
Your mission is "move down the ladder."

Why visceral fat is such a big deal for blood sugar

Visceral fat is like a noisy neighbor who throws trash directly into your liver's driveway.

Here is what tends to happen:

- Visceral fat releases fatty acids more easily.
- Those fatty acids drain straight to the liver through the portal circulation.
- The liver becomes more insulin resistant.
- The liver exports more VLDL, raising triglycerides.
- The liver leaks more glucose into the blood.

This is why someone can look "not that big," but have a high waist-to-height ratio and still struggle with prediabetes.

Visual: visceral vs subcutaneous (illustration)

Visceral fat

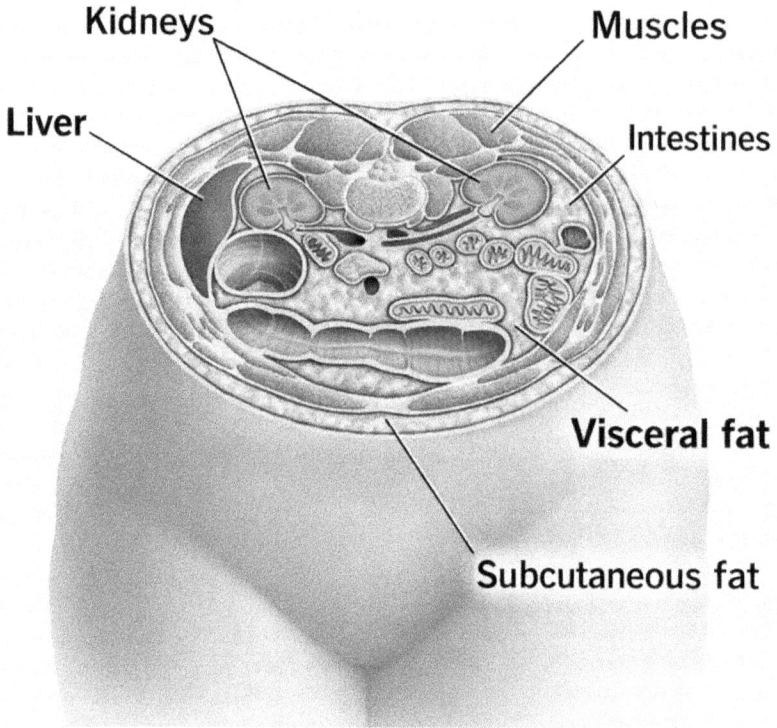

Subcutaneous fat is outside the muscle wall.

Visceral fat is inside, hugging organs.

One is mostly storage.

The other is storage plus metabolic trouble.

Actionables: reduce visceral fat, reduce risk

Here is the cool part: visceral fat tends to respond strongly when you fix the liver bottleneck and lower insulin levels.

1) Keep Step 4 levers consistent

From Chapter 9:

- cut sugary drinks
- reduce refined carbs
- use a consistent eating window

These target the liver. When the liver calms down, visceral fat often follows.

Time-restricted eating and intermittent strategies have shown improvements in liver fat and metabolic markers in MASLD studies, though protocols differ. (ScienceDirect)

2) Add one "muscle signal" each day

Muscle is a glucose sponge. You want more of it and you want to use it.
Pick one:

- 10-minute walk after your biggest meal
- 3 sets of squats to a chair
- pushups on a wall or counter
- light dumbbell rows with a backpack

This is not "gym culture." This is organ support.

3) Sleep protects your waist

Bad sleep increases hunger signals and worsens insulin sensitivity in many people, which makes visceral fat harder to drop.

Aim for:

- consistent bedtime
- phone away 30 minutes earlier
- a darker room

Not perfect. Just better.

4) Stop the "late-night second dinner"

If your eating window ends, it ends.

Late-night snacks are usually:

- sugar + refined carbs
- eaten when you are tired
- stored more easily because you are not moving

Make it boring:

- brush teeth
- peppermint tea
- go do something that uses your hands

"But I'm not that overweight" and other myths that steal progress

Myth 1: BMI tells the whole story.

BMI misses fat location. Waist helps reveal the risk you cannot see. (Obesity Canada)

Myth 2: Only older people get metabolic problems.

Central fat and fatty liver are showing up younger and younger, especially with high-sugar diets. (The Lancet)

Myth 3: If I lose weight, my health automatically improves.

Weight loss helps, but where you lose from matters. A smaller waist often signals a bigger improvement in metabolic risk than the same pounds lost elsewhere.

The "visceral fat reduction = risk reduction" explanation

Think of visceral fat like gasoline stored next to a fire.

Reducing it tends to:

- lower liver fat pressure
- improve insulin sensitivity
- improve triglycerides and HDL patterns
- reduce the metabolic syndrome cluster

And because cardiovascular disease is a major risk linked with fatty liver and metabolic dysfunction, this is not just about "numbers." It is about protecting your future. (AHA Journals)

Closing: one tape measure, real feedback

If you do nothing else this week, measure your waist correctly and write it down.

Not because you need another thing to worry about.

Because you finally deserve a metric that tells the truth about what is happening **inside**.

Next, we are going to take this a step further and talk about the lever that makes all of this easier or harder depending on how you use it:

insulin timing.

Not just "insulin is high," but *when* it stays high, *why* it stays high, and how to bring it down without feeling like your life is a punishment.

STEP 5: What NOT to do?

Insulin Injection Isn't the Fix

Uplifting fact: It is possible for many people with type 2 diabetes to reach normal-range A1C without insulin, and sometimes without any diabetes meds at all, when the root cause is addressed. (Diabetes Journals)

Let's start with a scene that feels way too real.

You go to a doctor. Your blood sugar is high. You are scared, because high sugar sounds like your body is "breaking." You want the number to come down fast. So the most obvious tool shows up: **insulin**.

And insulin works. It can pull glucose out of your bloodstream like a powerful vacuum.

But here's the problem.

Lowering sugar is not the same thing as fixing type 2 diabetes. It is like mopping the floor while the sink is still overflowing.

Remember the faucet analogy from earlier: if the faucet is blasting and the drain is narrow, the room floods. Exercising a bit is like widening the drain slightly. Helpful, but not enough if the faucet is still on full blast. The real solution is turning down the faucet.

In type 2 diabetes, the "faucet" is often **a steady stream of carbs and sugar feeding a system that is already overfilled.** The "overflow" is glucose and fat piling up in places they do not belong, especially the liver. That liver fat is strongly tied to insulin resistance and the whole diabetes spiral. (PubMed)

Why insulin can backfire in type 2

Insulin is a storage hormone. That is not an insult. It is its job description.

When you take insulin from the outside (as a shot), you are telling your body, "Store more. Push fuel into cells. Pack it away."

So yes, blood sugar drops. But for many people with type 2, **the suitcase is already overpacked.**

The overpacked suitcase analogy

Imagine you are trying to close a suitcase that is stuffed with clothes.

- Blood sugar is spilling out like socks popping through the zipper.
- Insulin is you pushing down on the suitcase lid with both hands.

You can sometimes get it shut. The outside looks "better." But inside, nothing became lighter. Nothing got organized. You just crammed harder.

And here's the kicker: when you cram harder, you often create a new problem.

Many people gain weight on insulin therapy. Not everyone. Not always. But it is common enough that it is a known issue in research and clinical practice. (PMC)

Why weight gain happens can be painfully simple:

- When sugar is high, some calories are literally lost in the urine.
- When insulin lowers sugar, those calories stay in your body.
- Insulin also tells the body to store energy, not burn it.

So if your strategy is "more insulin forever," you may lower the number while silently increasing the overflow that caused the number in the first place.

Luckily GLP-1's are recommended first now before starting insulin, unless there is a contraindication. GLP-1 receptor agonists offer significant benefits for people with type 2 diabetes by improving both **blood sugar control and weight management**. These medications work by enhancing glucose-dependent insulin secretion, suppressing excess glucagon, slowing gastric emptying, and increasing satiety—leading to meaningful A1C reductions with a **low risk of hypoglycemia** when used without insulin. In addition, GLP-1s consistently support **clinically significant weight loss**, which can further improve insulin resistance, cardiometabolic risk, and overall diabetes outcomes. Because of these advantages, current diabetes guidelines from the **American Diabetes Association** recommend considering a GLP-1 receptor agonist **before initiating insulin therapy** in many patients with type 2 diabetes, particularly those who would benefit from weight loss or have established cardiovascular risk. This approach reflects a shift toward therapies that treat both hyperglycemia and its underlying drivers, rather than focusing on glucose alone.

The "number-chasing" trap

Type 2 diabetes care can drift into something that looks responsible but can become misguided:

- A1C rises.
- Add a medication.
- A1C rises again.
- Increase medication.
- Repeat, until insulin is high, weight is higher, and the person feels like a failure.

But the failure is not the person. The failure is the strategy.

This is exactly the kind of logic Dr. Sarah Hallberg challenged when she said reversing type 2 diabetes starts with questioning the usual playbook. Her message hit millions because it matched what people were experiencing: the "standard" approach often did not feel like real healing. (YouTube)

Important nuance: insulin is sometimes necessary

This chapter is **not** "insulin is evil."

Insulin can be lifesaving, and sometimes it is the safest option:

- Very high blood sugar at diagnosis (for example A1C over 10% or glucose around 300 mg/dL).
- Symptoms of severe hyperglycemia like weight loss, dehydration, vomiting, confusion.
- Acute illness, surgery, pregnancy, or steroid treatment.
- When other meds are not enough or not safe. (Diabetes Journals)

The critique is about **strategy**.

If the long-term plan is only "push sugar down with insulin" while the root cause keeps growing, that is symptom control, not a reset.

What the big trials warn us about

One reason this matters is that "lower A1C at any cost" does not always lead to better outcomes.

In the ACCORD trial, intensive glucose lowering to near-normal A1C increased mortality and did not significantly reduce major cardiovascular events during the trial period. That result shocked a lot of clinicians and patients. (New England Journal of Medicine)

Other large trials (ADVANCE and VADT) showed mixed results: some microvascular benefits, but no clean story that aggressive glucose chasing guarantees heart protection for everyone. (New England Journal of Medicine)

Translation for real life:

- **Numbers matter.**
- **But numbers are not the whole story.**
- The goal is not just to score a better lab report. The goal is to get your body out of overflow.

Actionables: how to use insulin wisely if you need it

If you are on insulin now, here is a root-cause-friendly way to think:

1. **Use insulin as a safety tool, not as proof you are "broken."**
2. **Ask what is driving the overflow.** Food pattern, liver fat, sleep, stress, ultra-processed carbs, sugary drinks.
3. **Build an exit strategy when possible.** That might mean carb reduction, supervised fasting, weight loss, or newer meds that help reduce weight and insulin levels rather than raise them.

Patient empowerment script: questions to ask your clinician

Bring this like a calm, respectful checklist. You are not picking a fight. You are asking for a plan that makes sense.
Ask:

1. "What do you think is driving my high blood sugar: insulin deficiency, insulin resistance, or both?"
2. "If I start insulin, what is the plan to prevent weight gain and avoid rising doses?"
3. "Can we use a continuous glucose monitor or structured finger checks so I can see what foods spike me?" (PMC)
4. "Are there options that lower glucose while also helping with weight or insulin resistance?"
5. "What would remission mean in my case, and what milestones would show we are moving toward it?"
6. "If I change my diet quickly, how do we prevent low blood sugar?"
7. "What are my red-flag symptoms for hypoglycemia, and what is my exact plan if it happens?"

Safety

- **Never** stop insulin suddenly without medical guidance.
- If you are lowering carbs or experimenting with fasting, you must coordinate medication changes. Hypoglycemia is real, and it can be dangerous.
- If you have type 1 diabetes or you are unsure which type you have, insulin is not optional.

Curiosity for what's next: Insulin is the most powerful sugar-lowering tool, but it is not the only one. Next, we'll talk about pills and injections that can help, and how to tell whether a medication is acting like a "bandage" or like a lever that actually reduces overflow.

Pills: Tool, Not Cure

Uplifting fact: The right medication, used at the right time, can protect organs and buy you time while you fix the root cause, and some meds do this with less weight gain and less hypoglycemia than older options. (PubMed)

Let's talk about oral drugs and non-insulin injectables in a way most people never hear:

Meds can be useful tools.

But a tool is not automatically a cure.

A hammer can build a house. It can also smash your thumb if you do not know what it is doing.

Two categories that change everything

Most diabetes drugs fall into one of two "effects":

1. **Moves glucose around** (symptom-focused)
2. **Reduces overflow** (root-cause-aligned)

Some meds do a bit of both.

Here is the simplest mental model:

- If a medication mainly forces your body to make more insulin or store more fuel, it can lower glucose without reducing the underlying overload.
- If a medication helps your body become more insulin-sensitive, lowers liver fat, reduces appetite, increases glucose loss, or supports weight loss, it can be more aligned with reversal.

A quick, easy-to-understand map of common meds

Diabetes affects multiple systems throughout the body, which is why treatment often requires medications that work in **different physiological pathways** rather than a single solution. Blood sugar regulation involves at least **eight key areas**: the **pancreas** (impaired insulin secretion and excess glucagon), **liver** (overproduction of glucose), **muscle** (reduced glucose uptake), **fat tissue** (increased insulin resistance and free fatty acid release), **gut** (reduced incretin effect and altered nutrient signaling), **kidneys** (increased glucose reabsorption), **brain** (disrupted appetite and satiety signaling), and the **immune/inflammatory system** (chronic low-grade inflammation that worsens insulin resistance). Because diabetes impacts so many interconnected systems, **one medication alone is often not enough** to achieve optimal control. Many people need **multiple medications that target different organs and mechanisms** to lower blood sugars more effectively, improve insulin sensitivity, reduce complications, and create a more balanced, individualized treatment plan.

The good news is that because diabetes is affected by many parts of the body, there are many ways to improve it. Medicines help, but working on the root causes can help even more, like lowering fat stored in the liver, cutting back on sugary drinks and foods made with added sugars (including fructose), and choosing meals that keep you full. Some people also do well with time restricted eating or fasting if they can stick with it and their doctor says it is safe.

Metformin

Metformin is the classic first-line med for a reason. It improves insulin sensitivity and has strong outcome data from UKPDS showing benefit in overweight patients, with less weight gain and fewer hypoglycemic episodes than insulin or sulfonylureas. (PubMed)
How it often feels: gentle support, not a bulldozer.

Sulfonylureas (like glipizide, glyburide)

These push the pancreas to release more insulin.
They can drop glucose, but they are linked with **weight gain and higher hypoglycemia risk**, especially compared to many newer classes. (PMC)
This is "pack the suitcase harder" energy.

TZDs (like pioglitazone)

They can improve insulin sensitivity, but they can also cause fluid retention and weight gain, and they are not for everyone, especially people at risk for heart failure. (NCBI)

SGLT2 inhibitors (like empagliflozin, dapagliflozin)

These help the kidneys spill some glucose into urine. They also show cardiovascular and kidney benefits in many trials and meta-analyses. (PMC)
This is one reason modern guidelines increasingly emphasize protecting heart and kidneys, not just lowering glucose. (Diabetes Journals)

GLP-1 receptor agonists (like semaglutide)

Often reduce appetite, support weight loss, and improve glucose control. Trials and news coverage highlight broader cardio-renal protection and ongoing research. (Reuters)

The progression problem: treating numbers while overflow grows

This part is where people get angry, and honestly, they should.

If a treatment plan only aims to "hit the A1C target" but does not shrink the overflow, you can get this sad pattern:

- More meds
- More insulin
- More weight
- More insulin resistance
- More meds

It is not because the person is weak. It is because the plan is fighting biology.

This is why the old-school low-fat, high-carb approach was so devastating for many patients. It told people to eat more of the foods that raise glucose the most, then tried to medicate the spikes away. (ResearchGate)

And the harshest example is what happened when motivated teens tried to "Eat Less, Move More" under intense support in the TODAY study era. The failure rates were still extremely high. (NATAP)

The lesson is not "lifestyle never matters." The lesson is: **wrong lifestyle advice plus symptom-only meds is a trap.**

Actionables: medication choices that match your lifestyle plan

Use this as a conversation starter with your clinician.

If you are reducing carbs

Ask:

- "Can we lower or stop meds that cause hypoglycemia risk as my carbs drop?"
- "Do I need a CGM temporarily to stay safe during the change?" (PMC)

If you are doing time-restricted eating or fasting

Ask:

- "Which of my meds can cause low blood sugar on fasting days?"
- "What dose adjustments are planned in advance?"

A recent randomized trial of a 5:2 intermittent fasting meal–replacement approach showed improved glycemic control at 16 weeks in early type 2 diabetes, but any fasting strategy still requires smart medication supervision. (JAMA Network)

If weight loss is a primary lever for you

Ask:

- "Which meds support weight loss rather than weight gain?"
- "Can we prioritize cardio-renal protective meds if I have risk factors?"

"Medication + lifestyle" alignment checklist

Bring this list to your next visit.
For each medication I take, can my clinician tell me:

1. Does it mainly lower glucose today, or does it reduce insulin resistance

and overflow?

2. Does it increase insulin levels?
3. Does it commonly cause weight gain?
4. What is the hypoglycemia risk?
5. What happens to this med if I cut carbs or skip meals?
6. What is the plan to reassess in 8 to 12 weeks?
7. What is the long-term vision: management only, or remission attempt?

Safety

· Never change meds alone.
· Hypoglycemia risk rises when you combine carb reduction with insulin or insulin-stimulating drugs.
· Kidney function, blood pressure, and other conditions change what is safe.

Curiosity for what's next: Now that you can see the difference between "moves glucose" and "reduces overflow," we are ready for the big framework. The next chapter sorts strategies into reversal-supporting versus symptom-focused, and gives you a decision tree you can actually use.

Reversal vs Control

Uplifting fact: Major clinical research now uses the word **remission** for type 2 diabetes, defined as A1C under 6.5% for at least 3 months without glucose-lowering meds, because sustained reversal is real for a meaningful number of people. (Diabetes Journals)

Words matter. Here is the most freeing sentence you can learn in step 5:

Type 2 diabetes is not just a sugar problem. It is an overflow problem.

So the question becomes:

Are we draining the overflow, or are we just hiding it?

The cure vs no-cure framework

This is not a promise that everyone will get remission. It is a way to stop wasting effort on strategies that cannot logically work as a main plan.

Reversal-supporting strategies

These tend to reduce the overflow in the liver and pancreas, improve insulin sensitivity, and reduce the need for high insulin levels.

1. **Carb reduction, especially very low-carb for some**

- Many people see A1C improvement and medication reduction. (PubMed)

1. **Fasting or intermittent fasting (supervised if on meds)**

- Some trials and reviews show benefits, especially in early type 2 diabetes, but results vary and safety depends on meds. (JAMA Network)

1. **Substantial weight loss**

- In DiRECT, nearly half achieved remission at 1 year in the intervention group, and remissions tracked strongly with the amount of sustained weight loss. (The Lancet)

1. **Bariatric or metabolic surgery**

- Strong proof-of-mechanism because it often produces rapid glucose improvement and higher remission rates compared with medical therapy alone in selected patients. (PubMed)

Often symptom-focused when used alone

These can lower glucose, sometimes dramatically, but do not necessarily drain the overflow by themselves.

1. **Insulin escalation as the main long-term strategy**

- Can control glucose, but can add weight and higher insulin levels for some, and does not automatically reverse insulin resistance. (PMC)

1. **Insulin-stimulating drugs as the backbone**

- Can lower glucose but may raise insulin levels and bring hypoglycemia risk, often with weight gain. (PMC)

1. **Low-fat calorie restriction as the universal answer**

- Major trials like WHI and Look AHEAD did not show the promised cardiovascular win from the classic low-fat, calorie-reduced approach in broad populations. (JAMA Network)

Why the liver is the "quiet boss fight"

Many people are told, "Just exercise more."

Exercise is valuable. It improves muscle insulin sensitivity, blood pressure, mood, and more.

But here is the nuance: exercise cannot always fix the deepest part of type 2 diabetes on its own, because the liver component matters. Research on reversal and the twin cycle hypothesis emphasizes that excess liver fat drives hepatic insulin resistance and that improving this can happen quickly with significant dietary change and weight loss. (PubMed)

There is even research showing resistance training improved muscle insulin sensitivity without improving hepatic insulin resistance in a specific study context. That does not make exercise useless. It just shows why "exercise only" is rarely the full reset. (PMC)

"Choose your lever" decision tree

Use this as your personal map. Pick the lever you can actually pull consistently.
Step 1: Safety first

- If you are on insulin or sulfonylureas, do not fast or slash carbs without supervision.
- If you have a history of eating disorders, fasting may be emotionally unsafe.
- If pregnant, different rules apply.

Step 2: Pick your main lever

1. **Carb lever:** "I will cut the foods that spike my glucose."

- Best for people who like clear rules and quick feedback.

1. **Time lever:** "I will create longer breaks between eating."

- Best for people who snack constantly and want appetite freedom.

1. **Weight-loss lever:** "I will aim for meaningful weight loss with support."

- Best if you can access structured programs or meds that help appetite.

1. **Procedure lever:** "I want to discuss surgery as a metabolic reset."

- Best for people who meet criteria and want the strongest proof-of-mechanism option.

Step 3: Add a support lever

- CGM or structured glucose testing
- Sleep consistency
- Strength training
- Stress downshifts
- A clinician who treats you like a partner

Visual: "Lowers glucose today" vs "Drains overflow long-term"

Bringing it home with a human story

Elena was 63 and terrified, not just of diabetes, but of what it was stealing from her future: her energy, her confidence, her independence. She had the full metabolic syndrome package, plus fatty liver markers. Then she switched her strategy from "manage the number" to "drain the overflow." She used a low-carb, healthy-fat approach and structured fasting. Within weeks, she stopped metformin. A year later, she was off blood pressure meds, her A1C was in the normal range, and her liver markers normalized.

Richard was 76 and carrying a heavier load: stroke history, kidney disease, atrial fibrillation. He had been told escalation was the path. Instead, with a low-carb plan and careful fasting structure, he stepped down from insulin and eventually off oral meds, with his A1C landing in a normal range without diabetes drugs.

These stories are emotional because they flip the script: **they stopped treating diabetes like a life sentence and started treating it like a process that can move backward.**

Safety

- "Remission" is not "invincible." Follow-up still matters. (PMC)
- Medication changes should be planned, not improvised.
- If you have long-standing diabetes, remission may be harder, but im-

provement is still worth chasing.

Curiosity for what's next: Step 6 is where we make this personal. You will learn how to build your own "blood sugar rules" based on what your body does, not what a pyramid poster tells you to eat.

STEP 6 - The Two-Lever Plan (What Actually Helps)

You do **not** need a hundred hacks. You need **two levers**.

Lever 1 decides how much sugar enters your body.

Lever 2 decides how fast your body burns the sugar you already stored.

Most people keep yanking the wrong lever: they try to "move more" while still drowning their liver in sweet drinks and refined carbs. They feel guilty, tired, and stuck.

This step is about getting unstuck with a plan simple enough to follow when life is loud.

Lever 1: Less Sugar

Chapter 14

Uplifting fact: Cutting added sugar and refined carbs can improve blood sugar fast, sometimes within days, because you are reducing the biggest "glucose flood" hitting your bloodstream. (Diabetes Journals)

Imagine your blood like a hallway in a school between classes. When the bell rings, the hallway fills. If the doors keep opening every 30 minutes, the hallway never clears. That is what constant added sugar and refined carbs do: they keep the hallway packed. Your insulin has to scream louder and louder just to push glucose into storage.

And the scary part is this: modern sugar is not just "dessert." It is breakfast cereal that tastes like candy, "healthy" granola bars, sweetened yogurt, fancy coffee drinks, sports drinks, sauces, and breads that act like cake once they hit your blood. Ultra-processed foods are also linked to higher type 2 diabetes risk in large meta-analyses. (PubMed)

Why added sugar and refined carbs hit so hard

Not all carbs behave the same. The problem is **speed and processing**.

- **Added sugar and refined starch** (white bread, pastries, most crackers, many cereals) digest quickly and raise blood glucose fast.
- High glycemic index and high glycemic load eating patterns are associated with a higher risk of type 2 diabetes in cohort research. (PubMed)
- Sugary drinks are uniquely risky because liquid sugar hits fast and does not make you feel full the way real food does. A major meta-analysis found higher sugar-sweetened beverage intake is associated with higher risk of type 2 diabetes and metabolic syndrome. (PubMed)

If you want a clean, practical rule: **Stop drinking sugar. Then stop eating "naked carbs."** (Carbs without protein, fiber, or fat beside them.)

Fructose callout: the liver connection

Here is the villain most people never meet face-to-face: **fructose overload**.

Fructose is handled largely by the liver. In controlled studies, high fructose intake (especially from sweetened beverages) increased **de novo lipogenesis** (fat-making in the liver), worsened blood lipids, decreased insulin sensitivity, and increased visceral fat. (JCI)

And when people cut fructose-heavy added sugars for even a short time, studies in youth with metabolic issues showed improvements in markers like liver fat and insulin-related measures, even when calories were held similar. (ScienceDirect)

Simple translation: **If your liver is already "sticky" with fat, drowning it in sweet drinks is like pouring grease on a clogged drain.**

The Sugar Exit Plan

You are not "quitting sugar." You are switching identities: from someone who gets ambushed by sugar to someone who controls it.

The 7-day exit plan (fast relief)

Goal: Stop the biggest glucose spikes without feeling like your life ended.
  Day 1-2: Beverage reset

  - Water, sparkling water, unsweetened tea, black coffee.
  - If you hate plain water: add lemon, cucumber, mint, or a splash of unsweetened herbal tea.
  - Rule: **No calories in drinks.** (Milk drinks count as food.) (PubMed)

Day 3-4: Breakfast detox

  - Replace refined cereals, pastries, and white toast-only breakfasts.Choose whole grains, fruits, lean protein and vegetables.
  - Choose one template:
  - Eggs + veggies + fruit or whole-grain toast
  - Greek yogurt (unsweetened) + berries + nuts
  - Cottage cheese + sliced tomato + olive oil + salt

Day 5-6: "One ingredient carb" rule

  - If you eat carbs, pick carbs that look like food:
  - potatoes, oats, beans, lentils, fruit, intact whole grains
  - Avoid "powdered carbs":
  - white flour foods, most chips, crackers, pastries

Day 7: Build your default plate

- Half plate: non-starchy veggies
- Quarter plate: protein
- Quarter plate: smart carbs (optional)
- Add a thumb of healthy fat (olive oil, nuts, avocado)

This is not perfection. This is **traction**.

The 30-day exit plan (deep change)

Goal: Lower average blood sugar, lower cravings, and make it feel normal.

Week 1: Remove liquid sugar

- Zero sugary drinks, including "juice cocktails."
- If you do juice, treat it like dessert, not hydration.

Week 2: Remove "sweet breakfast"

- No cereal, toaster pastries, pancakes, sweet coffee drinks.
- Replace with savory or protein-forward breakfasts.

Week 3: Reduce refined grains

- Swap white bread, white pasta, most crackers.
- Upgrade to: beans, lentils, oats, quinoa, brown rice, potatoes with skin.
- Keep portions realistic and pair with protein.

Week 4: Make sugar occasional, not daily

- Pick 2 "planned treats" per week, not random treats every day.
- Eat treats **after a real meal**, not alone. That slows the glucose spike.

Shopping list swaps (easy wins)

Swap these

- Sweetened yogurt → plain Greek yogurt + berries
- Sugary cereal → oats + cinnamon + nuts
- White bread → sprouted or whole-grain bread (or lettuce wrap)
- Chips → nuts, popcorn, roasted chickpeas
- Candy → fruit + peanut butter
- Bottled sauces → olive oil + vinegar + spices

Label traps (they look healthy, but bite)

- "Fat-free" usually means more sugar or starch.
- "Gluten-free" can still be refined carbs.
- "Organic cane sugar" is still sugar.
- "Fruit concentrate" is still sugar.
- Watch serving sizes: the label is often playing hide-and-seek.

Beverage rules (non-negotiable)

1. **Do not drink sugar daily.** (PubMed)
2. "Sports drinks" are candy water unless you are doing long, intense training.
3. "Diet" drinks are a separate debate. If they keep your sweet cravings alive, treat them like training wheels: useful short-term, not a forever identity.

Visual: Carb Quality Ladder

Move down the ladder as your default. You do not need to live at Level 5 forever. You just need to stop living at Level 1.

Level 1: Fast sugar (worst)

101

- Soda, energy drinks, sweet coffee drinks, candy

Level 2: Refined starch

- White bread, white pasta, white rice, pastries, most crackers, many cereals

Level 3: Starchy whole foods

- Potatoes, corn, brown or wild rice (portion matters)

Level 4: High-fiber carbs

- Beans, lentils, oats, intact whole grains

Level 5: Whole foods (best)

- Non-starchy Vegetables, whole fruit

Higher fiber and lower processing generally means slower glucose rise and better fullness.

Meal templates (copy-paste meals)

Template A: Protein + color + fat

- Chicken + salad + olive oil
- Tuna + cucumber + avocado
- Eggs + spinach + feta

Template B: Bowl that does not spike

- Greek yogurt + berries + chia + walnuts
- Chili made with beans + ground meat + veggies

- Lentil soup + side salad

Template C: "Smart carb" plate

- Salmon + broccoli + small portion of potatoes
- Turkey + mixed veggies + quinoa
- Tofu + stir-fry veggies + brown rice (small)

The point: You are not banning carbs. You are upgrading them and putting them in their place.

Curiosity for next chapter: Lever 1 stops new sugar from flooding in. But what about the sugar already stored in the liver and belly fat? That is where Lever 2 gets almost unfairly powerful.

Lever 2: Burn Stored Sugar

Chapter 15

Uplifting fact: Intermittent fasting is not magic. It is a schedule change that can lower insulin exposure and help your body tap stored fuel, and research shows it can improve insulin resistance markers in some people compared to daily calorie restriction. (PMC)

You already fast every day. You just call it "sleep." Intermittent fasting simply **extends the quiet time** when your body is not processing incoming food.

And that quiet time matters because insulin is not just a blood sugar "helper." Insulin is also a storage signal. Constant intake means constant signaling.

What fasting is (and what it is not)

Fasting: a voluntary period of no calories (or near-zero calories), often with water, tea, or black coffee.

Not fasting:

- "Just a little snack" every two hours
- Creamy coffee drinks
- Grazing all day

Fasting is not a punishment. It is a **pause**.

Why intermittency matters

Here is the trap: people try to lose weight by cutting a small amount of food every day, forever. That can feel like living your whole life slightly hungry. It often triggers compensation: more cravings, less spontaneous movement, and your body trying to save energy. The Biggest Loser follow-up showed long-term metabolic adaptation after aggressive calorie restriction and weight loss, with resting metabolism remaining suppressed years later. (PMC)
Intermittency changes the pattern.

- Daily restriction: insulin goes down a bit, then stalls.
- Intermittent fasting: insulin gets real low for longer windows, giving the body time to use stored fuel.

In a randomized trial comparing alternate-day fasting to daily calorie restriction (with similar average weekly calories), the fasting pattern produced stronger improvements in insulin resistance markers in insulin-resistant participants. (PMC)

The hormonal advantages that constant intake blocks

When you eat all day, even "healthy snacks," you block the switch from storage mode to burn mode.
Fasting can shift hormones and signals in ways that constant intake often prevents, including:

- **Lower insulin exposure over time**, helping reduce insulin resistance

markers in some studies. (PMC)
- **Higher sympathetic activity** in early fasting, which may help explain why resting energy expenditure does not automatically crash in short fasting periods. (Nature)

You do not need to memorize hormones. You just need this image:
Constant eating = storage doors stay open
Fasting windows = storage doors finally close, burn doors open

History callout: fasting in diabetes care

Fasting is not new. In the pre-insulin era, physicians used severe carbohydrate restriction and undernutrition, including fasting, as one of the few tools available to manage diabetes, though it was harsh and controversial. (PMC)

Elliott P. Joslin published on diabetes treatment in 1916 in the *Canadian Medical Association Journal*, during a period when diet-based approaches were central. (PubMed)

And long before modern clinics, fasting showed up in spiritual practice for centuries, often described as a focused, disciplined reset. (You opened this step with that same ancient tone.)

Actionables: The Fasting Ladder

You do not jump from "late-night snacks" to a 36-hour fast. You climb.

Level 1: Start (12 to 14 hours)

Who this is for: almost everyone.

- Finish dinner, stop calories.
- Next day: breakfast later.
- Example: 8 pm to 10 am.

Win condition: You wake up and your first thought is not food panic.

Level 2: Standard (16:8)

Who this is for: people who feel stable on 12 to 14.

- Eat all meals within an 8-hour window.
- Example: 12 pm to 8 pm.

Pro tip: Keep the first meal protein-forward so you do not snap and hunt sugar at 3 pm.

Level 3: Advanced (24 hours)

Who this is for: people with experience who are not on high-risk meds.

- Dinner to dinner (or lunch to lunch) once per week.
- Hydrate well.
- Breakfast with a real meal, not a sugar bomb.

Level 4: Target protocol option (36 hours up to 3x/week)

Who this is for: advanced people, ideally supervised if medicated.

- Example pattern: dinner, fast next day, break following breakfast.
- This is powerful, but it is not casual.

What you can have during a fast

- Water (still or sparkling)
- Unsweetened tea
- Black coffee
- Electrolytes if needed (especially if you get headaches)

If you are fasting and you feel awful, do not "white-knuckle" it. Adjust the plan. Fasting is supposed to be challenging, not dangerous.

Safety: read this twice if you take diabetes meds

If you take **insulin or sulfonylureas**, do **NOT** start fasting without medical guidance. These medications are strongly linked to hypoglycemia risk during fasting periods. (NCBI)

Even the American Diabetes Association emphasizes hypoglycemia risk and recognizes symptoms like shakiness, sweating, confusion, and fast heartbeat. (American Diabetes Association)

Hypoglycemia warning signs checklist

If you feel any of these, check glucose if you can and treat per your clinician's plan:

- Shaky, trembling
- Sweating, chills, clammy skin
- Fast heartbeat
- Dizziness or lightheadedness
- Sudden hunger and nausea
- Irritable, anxious, confused
- Weakness, blurry visionSevere low blood sugar can cause seizures or loss of consciousness and is an emergency. (American Diabetes Association)

Safety mindset: It is safer to start with small fasting windows and adjust meds with a clinician than to improvise.

A simple "fasting day" script

· Morning: water, coffee or tea
· Midday: keep busy, salt your food on eating days, hydrate
· Evening (if eating): protein + vegetables first
· Sleep: earlier bedtime reduces snack temptation

Curiosity for next chapter: Fasting can feel like "surgery without surgery." Speaking of surgery, bariatric procedures can flip blood sugar fast. Why? And what can we learn from that even if you never go near an operating room?

Surgery Lessons

Chapter 16

Uplifting fact: Bariatric (metabolic) surgery can improve blood sugar rapidly, sometimes before major weight loss, because it changes fuel flow, liver glucose output, and gut hormones. (PMC)

Let's be real. Surgery is intense. It is not a "quick fix." But it teaches a brutally clear lesson:

When insulin drops and liver fat starts deflating, blood sugar can improve fast.

Why surgery can work quickly (beyond "calories")

There are two phases.

Phase 1: Immediate (days to weeks)

· Right after surgery, calorie intake drops hard.
· The liver reduces glucose output.
· Insulin sensitivity can improve quickly.
· A very-low-calorie diet can mimic some early improvements seen after Roux-en-Y gastric bypass in type 2 diabetes patients, suggesting the early

"magic" is strongly tied to rapid energy restriction and metabolic shifts, not only the anatomy change. (PMC)

Phase 2: Long-term (months to years)

- Significant fat loss changes insulin resistance.
- Gut hormones like GLP-1 increase after certain surgeries and can improve satiety and insulin response. (Diabetes Journals)

Who surgery helps (and who should pause)

Current guidelines recommend metabolic and bariatric surgery for people with higher BMI levels, and consider it for some people with metabolic disease at lower BMI ranges, depending on circumstances. (PMC)
Surgery can be life-changing for:

- Severe obesity with uncontrolled type 2 diabetes
- People who have tried structured medical therapy and still cannot control glucose safely
- People with serious obesity-related complications

But it also has real limits:

- It is still possible to relapse.
- Long-term remission rates vary, and recurrence after initial remission can happen. A 10-year follow-up paper reported complete remission in some patients, partial remission in others, and a meaningful rate of recurrence after initial remission. (PMC)

Surgery is a tool, not a personality transplant. It works best when behaviors change too.

Long-term considerations (the stuff TikTok forgets)

- Nutrition: protein targets, vitamins, minerals
- Follow-up: labs and check-ins
- Mental health: relationship with food often needs support
- Lifestyle: grazing on soft ultra-processed foods can still happen post-op

Actionables: "Surgery without surgery" principles

You cannot copy the anatomy. But you can copy the **principles** that make surgery powerful.

Principle 1: Create a real insulin break

This is fasting's superpower. If you constantly eat, insulin never truly rests. Controlled fasting windows can create low-insulin time.

- Start with 12 to 14 hours
- Build to 16:8 if tolerated
- Use 24-hour fasts occasionally if safe

Principle 2: Deflate the liver first

The liver is a key player in type 2 diabetes remission mechanisms after surgery. (PMC)

To deflate it without surgery:

- Stop liquid sugar
- Cut refined carbs
- Prefer whole foods carbs in smaller portions
- Prioritize protein and fiber

Principle 3: Change food form and order

After surgery, people often eat:

- smaller portions
- more protein first
- less ultra-processed snack food

You can copy that today:

- Eat protein and veggies first.
- Carbs last, if you want them.
- Avoid "melted calories" (chips, sweets, pastries) that disappear fast and do not fill you.

Principle 4: Make fullness easy

Surgery often increases satiety signals. You can support satiety with:

- protein at every meal
- fiber (veggies, beans, berries)
- healthy fats (olive oil, nuts)
- slower eating

Visual: Mechanism timeline (simple)

Day 1 to 7

- Calories drop hard
- Liver glucose output drops
- Blood sugar can improve quickly (PMC)

Week 2 to Month 6

- Appetite signals shift
- Weight and visceral fat often drop
- Insulin resistance improves

Month 6 to Year 10

- Maintenance decides the story
- Remission can persist, or recurrence can happen (PMC)

The big takeaway

Surgery screams the truth that our culture whispers around:

Type 2 diabetes is not only about willpower. It is about biology responding to food flow and insulin exposure.

And that is good news, because biology can change.

Curiosity for the next step: Now you have the two levers. Next comes the question that decides everything long-term: how do you keep this simple plan running during stress, social life, holidays, and the random Tuesday when motivation is dead?

STEP 7: Proof, Patterns, Prevention

Uplifting fact: Your body is not "bad at carbs." It is incredibly good at responding to the environment you give it.

Step 7 is about making this sustainable. Not "perfect." Not "all or nothing." Sustainable. Because the biggest trap is thinking you need one magic diet forever. You do not. You need a pattern that keeps insulin calm most days, and a simple reset when life gets messy.

In this step, you will see real-world proof (traditional diets), learn the maintenance default (Mediterranean, with a diabetes twist), and build a relapse-proof 90-day roadmap.

Chapter 17: Carb Context Matters

Uplifting fact: There are populations who eat high-carb diets and still have low fasting insulin and low rates of modern metabolic disease. That sounds impossible until you look at what "carbs" meant in their world. (PubMed)

The hook: why "carbs" is the wrong villain

If you have ever felt scared of a banana, confused by oatmeal, or angry because your friend eats pasta and "looks fine," you are not crazy. You are watching a word ("carbs") get blamed for a *context* problem.

Modern carbs are often:

- Pulverized (flour)
- Sweetened (added sugar, syrups)
- Liquid (soda, juice, fancy coffee)
- Designed for snacking (chips, bars, crackers)

Traditional carbs are often:

- Whole (tubers, fruit, beans)
- High in fiber and water
- Hard to overeat quickly
- Eaten as meals, not constant grazing

Same "macronutrient category." Totally different biological effect.

The Kitava reality check

Staffan Lindeberg and colleagues studied people on Kitava (Trobriand Islands, Papua New Guinea). Their diet was high in carbohydrate from whole foods like tubers and fruit, with minimal Western foods. Their fasting insulin levels were much lower than a Swedish comparison group, and body weight and blood pressure patterns looked strikingly different from modern industrialized norms. (PubMed)

Here is the point that matters for you:

High-carb did not automatically equal high insulin.

Low processing, low sugar-bomb foods, and a different eating rhythm changed the outcome.

The principle: processing + sugar + frequency beat "carbs"

If you want a simple mental model that actually works in real life:

1. **Processing:** Whole foods usually slow digestion and lower the insulin spike per bite. Ultra-processed foods push you to eat faster and more.

In controlled research, ultra-processed diets have been shown to drive higher calorie intake and weight gain compared with unprocessed diets, even when meals are designed to look "nutritionally matched" on paper. (PubMed)

2. **Sugar:** Added sugar is the "easy mode" for overeating because it is fast, sweet, and often liquid. It also sneaks into foods that pretend to be healthy.

3. **Frequency:** Constant snacking keeps insulin showing up like a group chat that never stops buzzing. Meal timing research suggests that *when* you eat can matter for diabetes risk, not just what you eat. (PubMed)

This is why two people can both say "I ate carbs" and get totally different outcomes.

Actionables: The "Carb Context Rules"

Use these as a simple filter, not a religion.

Rule 1: Whole-food carbs most days

Choose carbs that still look like something from nature:

- Potatoes, sweet potatoes, beans, lentils
- Fruit you chew (not juice you chug)
- Whole grains you recognize (oats, barley) if they work for you

Rule 2: Low sugar, especially liquid sugar

A sweet drink is a blood sugar shortcut.

- Soda, juice, energy drinks, sweet coffee drinks = "fast lane" glucose

Rule 3: Fewer eating episodes

Pick a meal rhythm you can live with:

- **2 to 3 meals** most days

115

· **Snacks only if planned**, and ideally protein-forward

Rule 4: "Carbs need a bodyguard"

If you eat a carb, pair it with:

· Protein (eggs, Greek yogurt, fish, chicken, tofu)
· Fiber (vegetables, beans)
· Healthy fat (olive oil, nuts, avocado)

This slows the rise and makes cravings quieter.

Visual: Carb Context Matrix

Think of insulin impact like a map:

EATING FREQUENCY

Intermittent Frequent

FOOD

Whole ✓ Best zone ⚠ Watch zone

(meals, whole) (constant grazing)

Refined ⚠ Risky zone ✗ Worst zone

(big spikes) (big spikes, all day)

Your goal is not "no carbs."

Your goal is to live in the **Best zone** as often as you can.

Bridge to the next chapter

Now that you know the real enemy is not "carbs" but *carb context*, you need a long-term pattern that makes this almost automatic. Next up: the Mediterranean approach, but tuned for lower insulin and real-world maintenance.

Chapter 18: Mediterranean, But Smarter

Uplifting fact: One of the most studied eating patterns in the world is not extreme, and it is strongly linked to heart protection, which matters because diabetes risk and heart risk travel together. (New England Journal of Medicine)

The hook: you do not need a "forever diet," you need a "default"

Most people fail because they try to white-knuckle a strict plan forever. That is like trying to hold your breath for life.

The Mediterranean pattern works as a default because it is:

- Flexible
- Social
- Built on real food
- Not obsessed with counting everything

In PREDIMED (a major randomized trial in Spain), a Mediterranean diet supplemented with extra-virgin olive oil or nuts reduced major cardiovascular events in high-risk adults compared with a control diet advice group. (New England Journal of Medicine)

And in a PREDIMED-related randomized trial focused on diabetes incidence, the Mediterranean diet supplemented with olive oil or nuts was associated with a lower incidence of type 2 diabetes compared with the control advice group (hazard ratios around 0.49 and 0.48 in the two Mediterranean groups). (PubMed)

Important honesty: these were mostly older, high-risk participants in Spain. Still, the pattern is powerful because the *mechanism* translates: fiber, fats, and protein anchors that reduce the chaos.

The diabetes twist: Mediterranean-Lower-Insulin

Classic Mediterranean can still go sideways if it turns into "bread with olive oil all day." So we tighten two screws:

1. **Protein anchor every meal (more chicken, fish, legumes, eggs, cheese, yogurt, nuts and seeds)**
2. **Vegetables first**
3. **Carbs are optional, and always contextual including whole grains and whole fruits**
4. **Good fats including more olive oil,olives, avocado, nuts, and seeds.**

Actionables: Meal templates

Use these like LEGO pieces.

Template A: Breakfast (choose 1)

- Eggs + spinach + olive oil, berries on the side
- Greek yogurt + nuts + cinnamon + a handful of berries + chia seeds
- Savory leftovers (yes, breakfast can be salmon and salad)

Template B: Lunch

- Big salad + chicken/tuna/tofu + olives + olive oil vinaigrette
- Lentil soup + side salad + feta
- Sardines on cucumber and tomato with olive oil and lemon

Template C: Dinner

- Fish + roasted vegetables + optional potatoes/beans
- Turkey/chicken bowl: veggies + olive oil + avocado + optional quinoa
- Stir-fry style Mediterranean: zucchini, peppers, mushrooms + protein + olive oil

Pantry build (your "maintenance toolbox")

Proteins: canned tuna/sardines, eggs, Greek yogurt, chicken, tofu
Fats: extra-virgin olive oil, olives, nuts, avocado
Fiber: frozen veggies, canned beans, lentils, berries, leafy greens
Flavor: garlic, lemon, vinegar, herbs, salt, pepper, chili flakes

Weekly plan (simple and repeatable)

- **2 fish meals**
- **2 poultry meals**
- **2 legume-based meals**
- **1 flexible meal** (social life meal)

That is it. No complicated math.

Visual: Mediterranean plate + anchors

Nutrition for Stabilizing
Blood Sugar

o VEG + FIBER

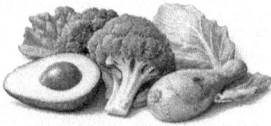

Brakes (slows glucose)

o [PROTEIN]

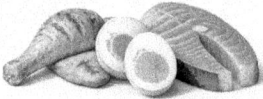

Stability
(less hunger)

o [HEALTHY FAT]

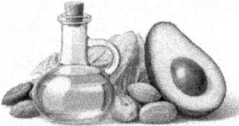

Satisfaction
(less craving)

Optional: [SMART CARB]

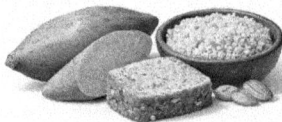

Only if it fits the moment

And the plate:

- Half plate: non-starchy vegetables
- Quarter: protein
- Quarter (or less): smart carbs, if you choose
- Olive oil (replaces butter) and nuts as the main fat

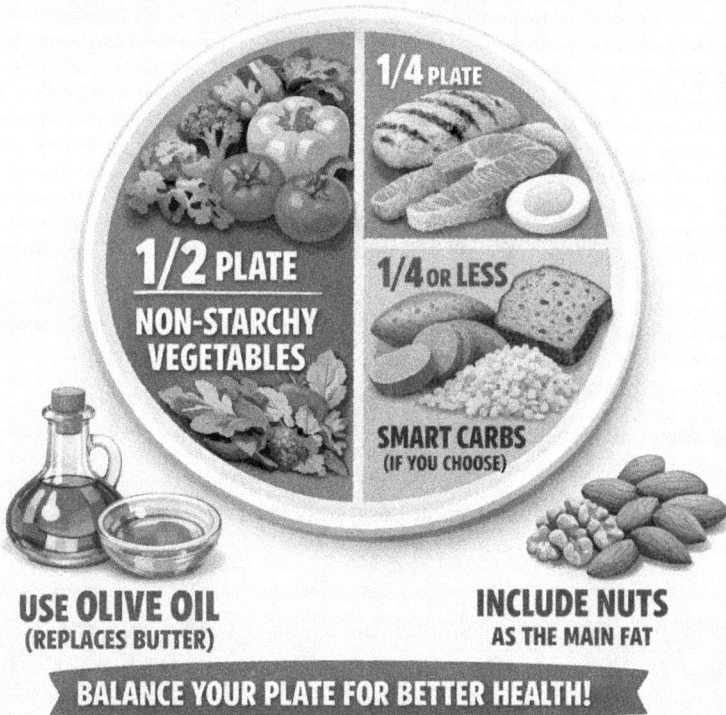

BUILD A HEALTHY PLATE

1/4 PLATE

1/2 PLATE
NON-STARCHY
VEGETABLES

1/4 OR LESS

SMART CARBS
(IF YOU CHOOSE)

USE OLIVE OIL
(REPLACES BUTTER)

INCLUDE NUTS
AS THE MAIN FAT

BALANCE YOUR PLATE FOR BETTER HEALTH!

Bridge to the next chapter

A good default still gets tested: holidays, breakups, exams, travel, "healthy" snacks that are secretly candy. Next you will build a 90-day system that keeps you in control even when life is not.

Chapter 19: The 90-Day Roadmap

Uplifting fact: Relapse is not a character flaw. It is usually a system problem. Fix the system, and your results stop feeling fragile.

Why relapse happens (the real reasons)

Relapse usually comes from one of these:

- **Holiday mode:** sugar everywhere, meals become snacks, snacks become meals
- **Stress:** you chase quick dopamine, and food companies know it
- **Sleep debt:** hunger hormones and cravings get louder
- **Travel:** airport food, weird schedules, "treat yourself" energy
- **The health halo trap:** granola bars, smoothies, low-fat flavored yogurt

Also, timing matters. Large cohort research has linked later first meals with higher type 2 diabetes incidence, suggesting the daily rhythm may shape risk. (PubMed)

You are not weak.

You are living in a world engineered for relapse.

Plateau troubleshooting (waist beats the scale)

If progress stalls, check in this order:

1. **Waist size** (visceral fat talks here first)
2. **Hidden sugars** (sauces, "healthy" snacks, drinks)
3. **Eating frequency** (are you in a constant nibble loop?)
4. **Protein too low** (you are hungry for a reason)
5. **Ultra-processed creep** (it sneaks in fast) (PubMed)

The 90-day plan (with milestones)

Weeks 1–2: Remove sugar + set meal rhythm

Goal: quiet the noise.

- Zero sugary drinks
- Dessert becomes "sometimes," not "daily"
- Choose **2 to 3 meals** most days
- Build meals with the anchors: protein, fiber, fat

Win marker: cravings shrink, energy steadies, you stop thinking about food every hour.

Weeks 3–6: Add the fasting ladder (gentle, safe)

Goal: create insulin "quiet time."

- Start with **12-hour overnight fast** (example: 8 pm to 8 am)
- If it feels good, move to **13 to 14 hours** a few days a week
- Optionally, try **16 hours** once or twice weekly if it fits your life

Safety note: if you use glucose-lowering meds or insulin, fasting can change your needs. Do not adjust medication alone.

Weeks 7-12: Personalize + lock maintenance

Goal: become your own coach.

- Pick your best carb context: which carbs work, which trigger cravings
- Decide your default week (Mediterranean-Lower-Insulin templates)
- Add a "tighten week" for when things drift

Win marker: you can travel, celebrate, and still return to baseline fast.

Tools

Weekly review template (10 minutes)

- What went well this week?
- What was the biggest trigger?
- Did I drink calories? (yes/no)
- How many days did I stick to 2–3 meals?
- Sleep average?
- Waist measurement (weekly, same day/time)
- One change for next week (make it small)

Lab discussion list (optional, but powerful)

If you choose to track markers with a clinician:

- A1c
- Fasting glucose
- Triglycerides and HDL (the ratio can be informative)
- ALT/AST (liver markers)
- Blood pressure

- Optional: fasting insulin (PubMed)

"Tighten vs loosen" rules

Tighten for 7 days if:

- Waist jumps up fast
- Cravings return hard
- Snacking becomes automatic
- Ultra-processed foods creep in daily

Loosen slightly if:

- You are consistent and stable for 3 to 4 weeks
- You can eat a smart carb and stop easily
- Sleep and stress are under control

Loosen does not mean "back to chaos."
It means "more flexibility inside the system."

Curiosity into what comes next

You now have proof, a default pattern, and a relapse plan. The next question is personal and powerful: **what kind of person do you become when blood sugar is no longer the boss of your day?**

Conclusion: your reset starts here

I f you made it this far, take a breath. You just did something important. You stopped accepting the old story that type 2 diabetes is a one way road that only gets worse.

You learned that type 2 diabetes is not a moral failure. It is not proof that you did not try hard enough. For many people, it is a predictable response to a modern food environment.

You also learned something hopeful. When type 2 is mostly driven by diet and lifestyle, then it can often be improved, and for many people it can reach remission.

What you learned in this reset

You learned that high blood sugar is not the root problem. It is a signal. The deeper issue is overflow.

Your blood is the hallway. Your cells are the rooms. Glucose is the delivery. Insulin is the key. In type 2 diabetes, the rooms are already full. When the rooms are full, the body resists taking more in. Blood sugar rises because glucose stays in the hallway.

That is why simply adding more insulin or more drugs without changing the input can control numbers without fixing the cause.

You learned why "eat less, move more" often fails in real life. Your body adapts. When you cut calories, energy use can drop. That is why willpower alone is not a plan. You need a strategy that works with biology, not against it.

You learned that this is not only about calories. It is about signals. Insulin is a major storage signal. Constant added sugar, refined starch, and constant snacking keep insulin high and keep the body in storage mode.

You learned that the liver matters. Fatty liver often comes before type 2 diabetes. Added sugars and refined foods can push the liver toward storing and making more fat, which worsens insulin resistance.

You learned why waist size matters more than the scale for many people. Visceral fat is strongly linked to insulin resistance and metabolic risk.

You learned that food quality matters. Traditional diets that are high in whole food carbohydrates are not the same as a modern diet high in sugar and refined flour. The real pattern behind the epidemic is added sugar, refined starch, ultra processed foods, and constant eating.

What helps, in one clear framework

The foundation is simple.

Put less sugar in.

Burn stored sugar.

Everything else supports these two moves. Carbohydrate reduction can help many people. Intermittent fasting can help many people. Meaningful, sustained fat loss, especially liver and visceral fat loss, can help many people.

You do not need extremes. You need a plan you can follow. Consistency beats intensity.

How the cookbook makes this easy

Knowing the why is not enough. Most people struggle with the same problem.

What do I eat on a normal day when I am tired and busy?

That is why I created The 5 Ingredient Diabetic Diet Cookbook for Beginners.

It turns the reset principles into daily meals you can actually make.

Five ingredients, so shopping is simple.

About 30 minutes a day, so it fits real life.

Meals under 10 dollars, so it is affordable.

A 60 day meal plan, so you do not have to decide every day.

This is not about perfect eating. It is about removing friction so you can repeat the right choices.

You can check it out here:

$$link

And whether you grab it today or simply take what you've learned and start making small changes right now, I want you to remember this:

You are not behind.

You are not broken.

You're choosing a different path.

That is what a reset is.

And it starts with the next meal and I truly wish you progress in the right direction.

A Quick Blessing

Your feedback is a true blessing!

If this book has encouraged you, helped you feel hopeful or gave you some useful tools, would you leave a quick review?

Even one sentence makes a huge difference and takes just a minute. As a small author, your feedback not only lifts my heart... It also helps others find the support and hope they need.

Thank you for being part of this journey!

Scan this QR code with your phone to go to the review page

Or

Go to your orders, find the book and click

"Write a product review"

Thank you <3

References (APA)

American Diabetes Association. (2025). *How type 2 diabetes progresses.* American Diabetes Association. (American Diabetes Association)

Bajahzer, M. F., et al. (2022). Effects of sugar-sweetened soda on plasma saturated and monounsaturated fatty acids. *[Abstract].* PubMed. (PubMed)

Bagust, A., & Beale, S. (2003). Deteriorating beta-cell function in type 2 diabetes: A long-term model. *QJM: An International Journal of Medicine, 96*(4), 281–288. (OUP Academic)

Carlsson, L. M. S., et al. (2012). Bariatric surgery and prevention of type 2 diabetes in Swedish obese subjects. *The New England Journal of Medicine.* (New England Journal of Medicine)

Estruch, R., et al. (2013). Primary prevention of cardiovascular disease with a Mediterranean diet. *The New England Journal of Medicine.* (New England Journal of Medicine)

Estruch, R., et al. (2018). Primary prevention of cardiovascular disease with a Mediterranean diet supplemented with extra-virgin olive oil or nuts. *The New England Journal of Medicine.* (New England Journal of Medicine)

Goldenberg, J. Z., et al. (2021). Efficacy and safety of low and very low carbohydrate diets for type 2 diabetes remission: Systematic review and meta-analysis. *BMJ, 372*, m4743. (BMJ)

Jayedi, A., et al. (2022). Anthropometric and adiposity indicators and risk of type 2 diabetes: A systematic review and dose-response meta-analysis. *BMJ, 376*, e067516. (BMJ)

Lindeberg, S., et al. (1999). Low serum insulin in traditional Pacific Islanders: The Kitava study. *[Abstract].* PubMed. (PubMed)

Lean, M. E. J., et al. (2018). Primary care-led weight management for remission of type 2 diabetes (DiRECT). *The Lancet.* (The Lancet)

Lean, M. E. J., et al. (2019). Durability of a primary care-led weight-management intervention for remission of type 2 diabetes (DiRECT): 2-year results. *The Lancet Diabetes & Endocrinology.* (PubMed)

Mazur, A. (2011). Why were "starvation diets" promoted for diabetes in the pre-insulin period? *Nutrition Journal.* (PubMed Central)

McFarlane, S. I. (2009). Insulin therapy and type 2 diabetes: Management of weight gain. *[Review].* PMC. (PubMed Central)

Ming, J., et al. (2015). Non-alcoholic fatty liver disease predicts type 2 diabetes mellitus. *[Abstract].* PubMed. (PubMed)

Most, J., et al. (2020). Impact of calorie restriction on energy metabolism in humans. *Physiology & Behavior / Review (PMC).* (PubMed Central)

Müller, M. J., et al. (2015). Metabolic adaptation to caloric restriction and subsequent refeeding. *The American Journal of Clinical Nutrition.* (ScienceDirect)

Pontiroli, A. E., et al. (2011). Increase of body weight during the first year of intensive insulin treatment in type 2 diabetes: Systematic review and meta-analysis. *Diabetes, Obesity and Metabolism.* (PubMed)

Sharma, S. K., et al. (2023). Intermittent fasting and type 2 diabetes glycaemic control: Systematic review/meta-analysis. *[PMC].* (PubMed Central)

Softic, S., et al. (2016). Role of dietary fructose and hepatic de novo lipogenesis in fatty liver disease. *Digestive Diseases and Sciences / Review (PMC).* (PubMed Central)

Stanhope, K. L., et al. (2009). Consuming fructose-sweetened, not glucose-sweetened, beverages increases visceral adiposity and decreases insulin sensitivity. *The Journal of Clinical Investigation.* (JCI)

Volk, B. M., et al. (2014). Effects of step-wise increases in dietary carbohydrate on de novo lipogenesis and triglycerides. *PLOS ONE.* (PLOS)

World Health Organization. (2016). *Global report on diabetes.* WHO. (World Health Organization)

Xu, F., et al. (2024). Fat distribution and diabetes in U.S. adults by race. *Frontiers in Public Health.* (frontiersin.org)

American Diabetes Association. (2013). *Economic costs of diabetes in the U.S.*

in 2012. Diabetes Care, 36(4), 1033–1046. https://pubmed.ncbi.nlm.nih.gov/23468086/

American Diabetes Association. (2021, August 30). *International experts outline diabetes remission diagnosis criteria.* https://diabetes.org/newsroom/international-experts-outline-diabetes-remission-diagnosis-criteria

Hall, K. D., Ayuketah, A., Brychta, R., et al. (2019). Ultra-processed diets cause excess calorie intake and weight gain: An inpatient randomized controlled trial of ad libitum food intake. *Cell Metabolism, 30(1),* 67–77.e3. https://pubmed.ncbi.nlm.nih.gov/31105044/

Himsworth, H. P. (2013). Diabetes mellitus: Its differentiation into insulin-sensitive and insulin-insensitive types (1936). *International Journal of Epidemiology, 42(6),* 1594–1598. https://pubmed.ncbi.nlm.nih.gov/24415598/

Imamura, F., O'Connor, L., Ye, Z., et al. (2015). Consumption of sugar sweetened beverages, artificially sweetened beverages, and fruit juice and incidence of type 2 diabetes: Systematic review, meta-analysis, and estimation of population attributable fractions. *BMJ, 351,* h3576. https://www.bmj.com/content/351/bmj.h3576

Karamanou, M., Protogerou, A., Tsoucalas, G., Androutsos, G., & Poulakou-Rebelakou, E. (2016). Milestones in the history of diabetes mellitus. *World Journal of Diabetes, 7(1),* 1–8. https://pmc.ncbi.nlm.nih.gov/articles/PMC4707300/

Lean, M. E. J., Leslie, W. S., Barnes, A. C., et al. (2018). Primary care-led weight management for remission of type 2 diabetes (DiRECT): An open-label, cluster-randomised trial. *The Lancet, 391(10120),* 541–551. https://www.thelancet.com/journals/lancet/article/PIIS0140-6736%2817%2933102-1/fulltext

Parker, E. D., Lin, J., Mahoney, T., et al. (2024). Economic costs of diabetes in the U.S. in 2022. *Diabetes Care.* https://pubmed.ncbi.nlm.nih.gov/37909353/

Piernas, C., & Popkin, B. M. (2010). Snacking increased among U.S. adults between 1977 and 2006. *The Journal of Nutrition, 140(2),* 325–332. https://pmc.ncbi.nlm.nih.gov/articles/PMC2806886/

Riddle, M. C., Cefalu, W. T., & Evans, P. H., et al. (2021). Definition and interpretation of remission in type 2 diabetes: Consensus report. *Diabetes*

Care, 44(10),

Browning, L. M., Hsieh, S. D., & Ashwell, M. (2010). A systematic review of waist-to-height ratio as a screening tool for the prediction of cardiovascular disease and diabetes: 0.5 could be a suitable global boundary value. *Nutrition Research Reviews, 23*(2), 247–269. (PubMed)

Church, T. J., & Haines, S. T. (2016). Treatment approach to patients with severe insulin resistance. *Diabetes Spectrum, 29*(2), 91–100. (PubMed Central)

Corkey, B. E. (2012). Banting Lecture 2011: Hyperinsulinemia: Cause or consequence? *Diabetes, 61*(1), 4–13. (PubMed Central)

Del Prato, S., Leonetti, F., Simonson, D. C., Sheehan, P., Matsuda, M., & DeFronzo, R. A. (1994). Effect of sustained physiologic hyperinsulinaemia and hyperglycaemia on insulin secretion and insulin sensitivity in man. *Diabetologia.* (Springer Link)

Furnica, R. M., et al. (2018). A severe but reversible reduction in insulin sensitivity is observed in insulinoma patients. *Clinical Endocrinology.* (PubMed)

Gregory, J. M., et al. (2019). Iatrogenic hyperinsulinemia, not hyper-glycemia, drives insulin resistance in type 1 diabetes. *Diabetes, 68*(8), 1565–1575. (Diabetes Journals)

Lean, M. E. J., et al. (2018). Primary care-led weight management for remission of type 2 diabetes (DiRECT): An open-label, cluster-randomised trial. *The Lancet, 391*(10120), 541–551. (The Lancet)

Lean, M. E. J., et al. (2019). Durability of a primary care-led weight-management intervention for remission of type 2 diabetes: 2-year results of the DiRECT trial. *The Lancet Diabetes & Endocrinology.* (PubMed)

Ross, R., Neeland, I. J., Yamashita, S., et al. (2020). Waist circumference as a vital sign in clinical practice: A consensus statement. *Nature Reviews Endocrinology.* (PubMed Central)

Smith, S. C., Jr. (2007). Abdominal obesity: Waist circumference as a more accurate predictor of cardiometabolic risk than BMI. *American Journal of Medicine.* (PubMed)

Taylor, R. (2021). Nutritional basis of type 2 diabetes remission. *BMJ, 374,* n1449. (BMJ)

Taylor, R. (2025). The twin cycle hypothesis of type 2 diabetes aetiology. *Diabetic Medicine.* (PubMed Central)

2438–2444. https://diabetesjournals.org/care/article/44/10/2438/138556 /Consensus-Report-Definition-and-Interpretation-of

Srour, B., Fezeu, L. K., Kesse-Guyot, E., et al. (2020). Ultraprocessed food consumption and risk of type 2 diabetes among participants of the NutriNet-Santé prospective cohort. *JAMA Internal Medicine, 180*(2), 283–291. https://pu bmed.ncbi.nlm.nih.gov/31841598/

U.K. Prospective Diabetes Study (UKPDS) Group. (1995). U.K. prospective diabetes study 16: Overview of 6 years' therapy of type II diabetes: A progressive disease. *Diabetes, 44*(11), 1249–1258. https://pubmed.ncbi.nlm.ni h.gov/7589820/

U.S. Department of Agriculture & U.S. Department of Health and Human Services. (1980). *Dietary guidelines for Americans (1st ed.).* https://www.dietar yguidelines.gov/sites/default/files/2019-05/1980%20DGA.pdf

World Health Organization. (2016). *Global report on diabetes.* https://www. who.int/publications/i/item/9789241565257

Wang, M., Yu, M., Fang, L., & Hu, R. Y. (2014). Association between sugar-sweetened beverages and type 2 diabetes: A meta-analysis. *Journal of Diabetes Investigation, 6*(3), 360–366. https://pmc.ncbi.nlm.nih.gov/articles/PMC442 0570/

U.S. Senate Select Committee on Nutrition and Human Needs. (1977/1978). *Dietary goals for the United States* (2nd ed.). https://www.govinfo.gov/content/ pkg/CPRT-95SPRT983640/pdf/CPRT-95SPRT983640.pdf

American Diabetes Association. (n.d.). *Diabetes diagnosis.* (American Diabetes Association)

American Diabetes Association. (2025). 2. *Diagnosis and classification of diabetes: Standards of care in diabetes 2025. Diabetes Care, 48*(Supplement_1), S27–S37. (Diabetes Journals)

Donath, M. Y., et al. (2022). Type 1 diabetes: What is the role of autoimmunity in β cell demise? *Journal of Clinical Investigation.*

(PubMed Central)

Hamman, R. F., et al. (2014). The SEARCH for Diabetes in Youth study: Rationale, findings, and future directions. *Diabetes Care.*

(PubMed Central)

Athanasaki, A., et al. (2022). Type 2 diabetes mellitus as a risk factor for Alzheimer's disease: Review and meta-analysis. Diabetes & Metabolic Syndrome: Clinical Research & Reviews. (PubMed Central)

Ciardullo, S., et al. (2023). Nonalcoholic fatty liver disease in patients with type 2 diabetes. *Journal of Clinical Medicine.* (PubMed Central)

Fox, C. S. (2010). Cardiovascular disease risk factors, type 2 diabetes, and the Framingham Heart Study. *Trends in Cardiovascular Medicine.* (PubMed Central)

Harding, J. L., et al. (2020). National and state-level trends in nontraumatic lower-extremity amputation. *CDC Stacks.* (CDC Stacks)

Holt, R. I. G., et al. (2024). Diabetes and infection: Review of the epidemiology and mechanisms. *Diabetologia.* (PubMed Central)

Holman, R. R., et al. (2008). 10-year follow-up of intensive glucose control in type 2 diabetes. *New England Journal of Medicine.* (New England Journal of Medicine)

UK Prospective Diabetes Study (UKPDS) Group. (1999). UKPDS and complications overview. *Diabetes Care* / review summaries. (PubMed Central)

World Health Organization. (2016). *Global report on diabetes.* (For broader context on complications and burden). (CDC)

Sources (APA)

Ashwell, M., & Gibson, S. (2014). *Waist-to-height ratio is more predictive of years of life lost than body mass index.* PLOS ONE. (PLOS)

Colditz, G. A., Willett, W. C., Rotnitzky, A., & Manson, J. E. (1995). Weight gain as a risk factor for clinical diabetes mellitus in women. *Annals of Internal Medicine,* 122(7), 481–486. (PubMed)

Fothergill, E., Guo, J., Howard, L., et al. (2016). Persistent metabolic adaptation 6 years after "The Biggest Loser" competition. *Obesity.* (PubMed)

Howard, B. V., Van Horn, L., Hsia, J., et al. (2006). Low-fat dietary pattern and weight change over 7 years: The Women's Health Initiative Dietary Modification Trial. *JAMA*. (JAMA Network)

Klein, S., Fontana, L., Young, V. L., et al. (2004). Absence of an effect of liposuction on insulin action and risk factors for coronary heart disease. *The New England Journal of Medicine*. (PubMed)

Knowler, W. C., Barrett-Connor, E., Fowler, S. E., et al. (2002). Reduction in the incidence of type 2 diabetes with lifestyle intervention or metformin. *The New England Journal of Medicine, 346*(6), 393–403. (New England Journal of Medicine)

Spiegel, K., Leproult, R., & Van Cauter, E. (1999). Impact of sleep debt on metabolic and endocrine function. *The Lancet*. (PubMed)

Tabák, A. G., Jokela, M., Akbaraly, T. N., Brunner, E. J., Kivimäki, M., & Witte, D. R. (2009). Trajectories of glycaemia, insulin sensitivity, and insulin secretion before diagnosis of type 2 diabetes: An analysis from the Whitehall II study. *The Lancet, 373*(9682), 2215–2221. (PubMed)

Wang, M., Yu, M., Fang, L., & Hu, R. Y. (2014). Association between sugar-sweetened beverages and type 2 diabetes: A meta-analysis. *Journal of Diabetes Investigation*. (PubMed Central)

Yaribeygi, H., Farrokhi, F. R., Butler, A. E., & Sahebkar, A. (2022). Molecular mechanisms linking stress and insulin resistance. *Journal of Cellular Physiology*. (PubMed Central)

Sources (APA)

Carpentier, A. C. (2021). Insulin and adipose tissue fatty acid metabolism. *American Journal of Physiology-Endocrinology and Metabolism*. (Physiology Journals)

Haber, R., et al. (2024). The impact of metformin on weight and metabolic parameters in adults: A systematic review and meta-analysis. *Diabetes, Obesity and Metabolism*. (dom-pubs.onlinelibrary.wiley.com)

Hemmingsen, B., et al. (2014). Sulfonylurea versus metformin monotherapy in patients with type 2 diabetes: A systematic review. *CMAJ Open, 2*(3),

E162–E175. (cmajopen.ca)

Kersten, S. (2001). Mechanisms of nutritional and hormonal regulation of lipogenesis. *EMBO Reports, 2*(4), 282–286. (PubMed Central)

McFarlane, S. I., et al. (2009). Insulin therapy and type 2 diabetes: Management of weight gain. *Diabetes, Metabolic Syndrome and Obesity.* (PubMed Central)

Pontiroli, A. E., et al. (2011). Increase of body weight during the first year of intensive insulin treatment in type 2 diabetes: Systematic review and meta-analysis. *Diabetes, Obesity and Metabolism.* (PubMed)

Sanders, F. W. B., & Griffin, J. L. (2016). De novo lipogenesis in the liver in health and disease: More than just a shunting yard for glucose. *Biological Reviews.* (Wiley Online Library)

Santoro, A., et al. (2021). Insulin action in adipocytes, adipose remodeling, and systemic effects. *Endocrine Reviews.* (PubMed Central)

Smith, G. I., et al. (2020). Insulin resistance drives hepatic de novo lipogenesis in nonalcoholic fatty liver disease. *Journal of Clinical Investigation.* (PubMed Central)

Taylor, R., et al. (2018). Remission of human type 2 diabetes requires decrease in liver and pancreas fat content but is dependent upon capacity for β cell recovery. *Cell Metabolism, 28*(4), 547–556.e3. (PubMed)

Yerevanian, A., & Shulman, G. I. (2019). Metformin: Mechanisms in human obesity and weight loss. *Current Obesity Reports.* (PubMed Central)

Zammit, V. A. (2001). Insulin stimulation of hepatic triacylglycerol secretion and lipid-related insulin resistance. *The Journal of Nutrition.* (sciencedirect.com)

Bird, S. R., & Hawley, J. A. (2017). Update on the effects of physical activity on insulin sensitivity in humans. *BMJ Open Sport & Exercise Medicine, 2*(1), e000143. https://pmc.ncbi.nlm.nih.gov/articles/PMC5569266/

Corkey, B. E. (2012). Banting Lecture 2011: Hyperinsulinemia: Cause or consequence? *Diabetes, 61*(1), 4–13. https://pubmed.ncbi.nlm.nih.gov/22187369/

Del Prato, S., et al. (1994). Effect of sustained physiologic hyperinsulinaemia and hyperglycaemia on insulin secretion and insulin sensitivity in man.

Diabetologia, 37, 1025–1035. https://link.springer.com/article/10.1007/BF0 0400466 (Springer Link)

Marangou, A. G., et al. (1986). Metabolic consequences of prolonged hyperinsulinemia in humans. *Diabetologia, 29*(11), 781–787. https://pubmed. ncbi.nlm.nih.gov/3533684/ (PubMed)

Manco, M., et al. (2017). Insulin resistance and NAFLD: A dangerous liaison. *International Journal of Molecular Sciences, 18*(7), 1597. https://pdfs.semanti cscholar.org/7888/215f3f6485beeb2950d2f6b2a0c72aefdbbd.pdf (Semantic Scholar)

Sattar, N., & Gill, J. M. R. (2014). Type 2 diabetes as a disease of ectopic fat? *BMC Medicine, 12,* 123. https://pmc.ncbi.nlm.nih.gov/articles/PMC4143560/ (pmc.ncbi.nlm.nih.gov)

Browning, L. M., Hsieh, S. D., & Ashwell, M. (2010). A systematic review of waist-to-height ratio as a screening tool for the prediction of cardiovascular disease and diabetes: 0.5 could be a suitable global boundary value. *Nutrition Research Reviews, 23*(2), 247–269. (Cambridge University Press & Assessment)

Dharmalingam, M., & Yamasandhi, P. G. (2018). Nonalcoholic fatty liver disease and type 2 diabetes mellitus. *Indian Journal of Endocrinology and Metabolism, 22*(3), 421–428. (PMC)

Jayedi, A., Soltani, S., Zargar, M. S., Khan, T. A., & Shab-Bidar, S. (2022). Anthropometric and adiposity indicators and risk of type 2 diabetes: Systematic review and dose-response meta-analysis of cohort studies. *The BMJ, 376,* e067516. (BMJ)

Lean, M. E. J., Leslie, W. S., Barnes, A. C., Brosnahan, N., Thom, G., McCombie, L., ... Taylor, R. (2018). Primary care-led weight management for remission of type 2 diabetes (DiRECT): An open-label, cluster-randomised trial. *The Lancet, 391*(10120), 541–551. (PubMed)

Randle, P. J., Garland, P. B., Hales, C. N., & Newsholme, E. A. (1963). The glucose fatty-acid cycle: Its role in insulin sensitivity and the metabolic disturbances of diabetes mellitus. *The Lancet, 281*(7285), 785–789. (PubMed)

Softic, S., Cohen, D. E., & Kahn, C. R. (2016). Role of dietary fructose and hepatic de novo lipogenesis in fatty liver disease. *Digestive Diseases and Sciences, 61*(5), 1282–1293. (PMC)

Schwarz, J. M., Noworolski, S. M., Erkin-Cakmak, A., Korn, N. J., Wen, M. J., Tai, V. W., ... Lustig, R. H. (2017). Effects of dietary fructose restriction on liver fat, de novo lipogenesis, and insulin kinetics in children with obesity. *Gastroenterology, 153*(3), 743–752. (Gastro Journal)

Taylor, R., Al-Mrabeh, A., Zhyzhneuskaya, S., Peters, C., Barnes, A. C., Aribisala, B. S., ... Lean, M. E. J. (2018). Remission of human type 2 diabetes requires decrease in liver and pancreas fat content but is dependent upon capacity for β cell recovery. *Cell Metabolism, 28*(4), 547–556.e3. (PubMed)

Imamura, F., O'Connor, L., Ye, Z., Mursu, J., Hayashino, Y., Bhupathiraju, S. N., & Forouhi, N. G. (2015). Consumption of sugar sweetened beverages, artificially sweetened beverages, and fruit juice and incidence of type 2 diabetes: Systematic review, meta-analysis, and estimation of population attributable fraction. *BMJ, 351*, h3576. (BMJ)

Mantovani, A., Byrne, C. D., Bonora, E., & Targher, G. (2018). Nonalcoholic fatty liver disease and risk of incident type 2 diabetes: A meta-analysis. *Diabetes Care, 41*(2), 372–382. (PubMed)

Rinella, M. E., Lazarus, J. V., Ratziu, V., Francque, S. M., Sanyal, A. J., Kanwal, F., Romero, D., Abdelmalek, M. F., Anstee, Q. M., Arab, J. P., et al. (2023). A multisociety Delphi consensus statement on new fatty liver disease nomenclature. *Journal of Hepatology.* (Journal of Hepatology)

Schwarz, J. M., Noworolski, S. M., Wen, M. J., Dyachenko, A., Prior, J. L., Weinberg, M. E., Herraiz, L. A., Tai, V. W., & Mulligan, K. (2017). Effects of dietary fructose restriction on liver fat, de novo lipogenesis, and insulin kinetics in children with obesity. *Gastroenterology.* (Gastro Journal)

Stanhope, K. L., Schwarz, J. M., Keim, N. L., Griffen, S. C., Bremer, A. A., Graham, J. L., Hatcher, B., Cox, C. L., Dyachenko, A., Zhang, W., et al. (2009). Consuming fructose-sweetened, not glucose-sweetened, beverages increases visceral adiposity and lipids and decreases insulin sensitivity in over-weight/obese humans. *The Journal of Clinical Investigation, 119*(5), 1322–1334.

(PubMed)

Sutton, E. F., Beyl, R., Early, K. S., Cefalu, W. T., Ravussin, E., & Peterson, C. M. (2018). Early time-restricted feeding improves insulin sensitivity, blood pressure, and oxidative stress even without weight loss in men with prediabetes. *Cell Metabolism, 27*(6), 1212–1221.e3. (PubMed)

Taylor, R. (2008). Pathogenesis of type 2 diabetes: Tracing the reverse route from cure to cause. *Diabetologia, 51*, 1781–1789. (Newcastle University)

Volk, B. M., Kunces, L. J., Freidenreich, D. J., Kupchak, B. R., Saenz, C., Artistizabal, J. C., Fernandez, M. L., & Volek, J. S. (2014). Effects of step-wise increases in dietary carbohydrate on circulating saturated fatty acids and palmitoleic acid in adults. *PLOS ONE, 9*(11), e113605. (PLOS)

Younossi, Z. M., Golabi, P., Paik, J. M., Henry, L., Van Dongen, C., & Henry, A. (2023). The global epidemiology of nonalcoholic fatty liver disease and nonalcoholic steatohepatitis: A systematic review. *Hepatology, 77*(4), 1335–1347. (PubMed)

Cesaro, A., et al. (2023). *Visceral adipose tissue and residual cardiovascular risk.* Frontiers in Cardiovascular Medicine. (Frontiers)

Jayedi, A., et al. (2022). Anthropometric and adiposity indicators and risk of type 2 diabetes. *BMJ, 376*, e067516. (BMJ)

Klein, S., et al. (2004). Absence of an effect of liposuction on insulin action and risk factors for coronary heart disease. *The New England Journal of Medicine, 350*(25), 2549–2557. (New England Journal of Medicine)

Kodama, S., et al. (2012). Comparisons of the strength of associations with future type 2 diabetes risk: Waist-to-height ratio, waist circumference, BMI, and waist-to-hip ratio. *Diabetologia.* (PubMed)

Merlotti, C., Ceriani, V., Morabito, A., & Pontiroli, A. E. (2017). Subcutaneous fat loss is greater than visceral fat loss with diet and exercise: A critical review and meta-analysis. *International Journal of Obesity, 41*, 672–682. (PubMed)

Reaven, G. M. (1988). Role of insulin resistance in human disease (Banting Lecture). *Diabetes, 37*(12), 1595–1607. (PubMed)

Reisinger, C., et al. (2021). The prevalence of pediatric metabolic syndrome. *International Journal of Obesity.* (Nature)

Sanguankeo, A., et al. (2016). Effects of visceral adipose tissue reduction on cardiovascular disease risk factors: A systematic review and meta-analysis. *Lipids in Health and Disease*. (PubMed Central)

Vissers, D., et al. (2013). The effect of exercise on visceral adipose tissue in overweight adults: A systematic review and meta-analysis. *PLOS ONE, 8*(2), e56415. (PLOS)

International Diabetes Federation. (2005). *The IDF worldwide definition of the metabolic syndrome.*

International Diabetes Federation. (2007). *The IDF consensus definition of metabolic syndrome in children and adolescents.*

Fothergill, E., Guo, J., Howard, L., Kerns, J. C., Knuth, N. D., Brychta, R., Chen, K. Y., Skarulis, M. C., Walter, M., Walter, P. J., & Hall, K. D. (2016). Persistent metabolic adaptation 6 years after "The Biggest Loser" competition. *Obesity, 24*(8), 1612–1619. (PubMed Central)

Goldenberg, J. Z., Day, A., Brinkworth, G. D., Sato, J., Yamada, S., Jönsson, T., Beardsley, J., Johnson, J. A., & Thabane, L. (2021). Efficacy and safety of low and very low carbohydrate diets for type 2 diabetes remission: Systematic review and meta-analysis of randomized trials. *BMJ, 372*, m4743. (BMJ)

Howard, B. V., Manson, J. E., Stefanick, M. L., Beresford, S. A. A., Frank, G., Jones, B., Rodabough, R. J., Snetselaar, L., Thomson, C., Tinker, L., Vitolins, M., Prentice, R., & Women's Health Initiative Investigators. (2006). Low-fat dietary pattern and weight change over 7 years: The Women's Health Initiative Dietary Modification Trial. *JAMA, 295*(1), 39–49. (PubMed)

Howard, B. V., Van Horn, L., Hsia, J., Manson, J. E., Stefanick, M. L., Wassertheil-Smoller, S., Kuller, L. H., LaCroix, A. Z., Langer, R. D., Lasser, N. L., Lewis, C. E., Limacher, M. C., Margolis, K. L., Mysiw, W. J., Ockene, J. K., Parker, L. M., Perri, M. G., Phillips, L., Prentice, R. L., … Women's Health Initiative Investigators. (2006). Low-fat dietary pattern and risk of cardiovascular disease: The Women's Health Initiative Randomized Controlled Dietary Modification Trial. *JAMA, 295*(6), 655–666. (PubMed)

Look AHEAD Research Group. (2013). Cardiovascular effects of intensive lifestyle intervention in type 2 diabetes. *The New England Journal of Medicine, 369*(2), 145–154. (New England Journal of Medicine)

Rosenbaum, M., & Leibel, R. L. (2010). Adaptive thermogenesis in humans. *International Journal of Obesity, 34*(Suppl 1), S47–S55. (PubMed)

Silva, A. M., Júdice, P. B., Carraca, E. V., King, N., Teixeira, P. J., & Sardinha, L. B. (2018). What is the effect of diet and/or exercise interventions on behavioural compensation in non-exercise physical activity and related energy expenditure of free-living adults? A systematic review. *British Journal of Nutrition, 119*(12), 1320–1330. (Cambridge University Press & Assessment)

Umpierre, D., Ribeiro, P. A. B., Kramer, C. K., Leitão, C. B., Zucatti, A. T. N., Azevedo, M. J., Gross, J. L., Ribeiro, J. P., & Schaan, B. D. (2011). Physical activity advice only or structured exercise training and association with HbA1c levels in type 2 diabetes: A systematic review and meta-analysis. *JAMA, 305*(17), 1790–1799. (JAMA Network)

Zeitler, P., Hirst, K., Pyle, L., Linder, B., Copeland, K., Arslanian, S., Cuttler, L., Nathan, D. M., Tollefsen, S., & TODAY Study Group. (2012). A clinical trial to maintain glycemic control in youth with type 2 diabetes. *The New England Journal of Medicine, 366*(24), 2247–2256. (New England Journal of Medicine)

Alberti, K. G. M. M., et al. (2006). Metabolic syndrome: A new worldwide definition. (Wiley Online Library)

International Diabetes Federation. (2007). *The IDF consensus worldwide definition of the metabolic syndrome.* (International Diabetes Federation)

Kassi, E., et al. (2011). Metabolic syndrome: Definitions and controversies. (PubMed Central)

Lin, X., et al. (2024). The effects of time-restricted eating for patients with NAFLD: A review. (PubMed Central)

Oh, J. H., et al. (2025). Efficacy and safety of time-restricted eating in MASLD: Randomized trial. (ScienceDirect)

Pinho, C. P. S., et al. (2018). Waist circumference measurement sites and association with visceral fat. (PubMed Central)

Ruano, G. R., et al. (2025). Abdominal obesity and cardiometabolic risk markers. (ScienceDirect)

Targher, G., et al. (2022). Nonalcoholic fatty liver disease and cardiovascular risk. *Arteriosclerosis, Thrombosis, and Vascular Biology.* (AHA Journals)

Wang, Y., et al. (2024). 5:2 intermittent fasting versus daily calorie restriction on hepatic steatosis. (Frontiers)

ADVANCE Collaborative Group. (2008). Intensive blood glucose control and vascular outcomes in patients with type 2 diabetes. *New England Journal of Medicine, 358*(24), 2560–2572. (New England Journal of Medicine)

American Diabetes Association. (2025). 9. Pharmacologic approaches to glycemic treatment: Standards of care in diabetes. *Diabetes Care, 48*(Supplement 1), S181–S206. (Diabetes Journals)

Bolli, G. B., et al. (2025). The modern role of basal insulin in advancing therapy in type 2 diabetes. *Diabetes Care, 48*(5), 671–684. (Diabetes Journals)

Croymans, D. M., et al. (2013). Resistance training improves indices of muscle insulin sensitivity and β-cell function but not hepatic insulin resistance. *Journal of Applied Physiology.* (PMC)

Dehghani, M., et al. (2024). Efficacy and safety of basal insulins in people with type 2 diabetes: A systematic review and network meta-analysis. *[PubMed record].* (PubMed)

Dyńka, D., et al. (2025). Intermittent fasting in the treatment of type 2 diabetes. *[Review, PMC].* (PMC)

Duckworth, W., et al. (2009). Glucose control and vascular complications in veterans with type 2 diabetes. *New England Journal of Medicine, 360*(2), 129–139. (New England Journal of Medicine)

Gerstein, H. C., et al. (2008). Effects of intensive glucose lowering in type 2 diabetes. *New England Journal of Medicine, 358*(24), 2545–2559. (New England Journal of Medicine)

Guo, L., et al. (2024). A 5:2 intermittent fasting meal replacement diet and glycemic control in adults with early type 2 diabetes: A randomized clinical trial. *JAMA Network Open.* (JAMA Network)

Hallberg, S. J. (2015). *Reversing type 2 diabetes starts with ignoring the guidelines* [TEDx Talk]. TEDxPurdueU. (YouTube)

Hallberg, S. J., et al. (2018). Effectiveness and safety of a novel care model for the management of type 2 diabetes at 1 year. *Diabetes Therapy, 9,* 583–612. (PubMed)

Howard, B. V., et al. (2006). Low-fat dietary pattern and risk of cardiovascular disease: The Women's Health Initiative randomized controlled dietary modification trial. *JAMA, 295*(6), 655–666. (JAMA Network)

Hu, F. B., et al. (1997). Dietary fat intake and the risk of coronary heart disease in women. *New England Journal of Medicine, 337*(21), 1491–1499. (PubMed)

Lean, M. E. J., et al. (2018). Primary care-led weight management for remission of type 2 diabetes (DiRECT). *The Lancet, 391*(10120), 541–551. (The Lancet)

Lean, M. E. J., et al. (2019). Durability of a primary care-led weight-management intervention for remission of type 2 diabetes: 2-year results (DiRECT). *The Lancet Diabetes & Endocrinology, 7*(5), 344–355. (PubMed)

Look AHEAD Research Group. (2013). Cardiovascular effects of intensive lifestyle intervention in type 2 diabetes. *New England Journal of Medicine, 369*(2), 145–154. (New England Journal of Medicine)

Marušić, M., et al. (2021). NAFLD, insulin resistance, and type 2 diabetes mellitus. *[Review, PMC].* (PMC)

Riddle, M. C., et al. (2021). Consensus report: Definition and interpretation of remission in type 2 diabetes. *Diabetes Care, 44*(10), 2438–2444. (Diabetes Journals)

Schauer, P. R., et al. (2017). Bariatric surgery versus intensive medical therapy for diabetes: 5-year outcomes (STAMPEDE). *New England Journal of Medicine, 376*(7), 641–651. (PubMed)

Taylor, R. (2013). Reversing the twin cycles of type 2 diabetes. *Banting Memorial Lecture* (PDF). (Newcastle University)

Taylor, R. (2021). Type 2 diabetes and remission: Practical management based on the twin cycle hypothesis. *[PubMed record].* (PubMed)

UK Prospective Diabetes Study (UKPDS) Group. (1998). Effect of intensive blood-glucose control with metformin on complications in overweight patients with type 2 diabetes. *The Lancet, 352*(9131), 854–865. (PubMed)

American Diabetes Association. (2025). *6. Glycemic goals and hypoglycemia: Standards of care in diabetes 2025. Diabetes Care, 48*(Supplement 1), S128-S145.

(Diabetes Journals)

American Diabetes Association. (2019). Nutrition therapy for adults with diabetes or prediabetes: A consensus report. *Diabetes Care, 42*(5), 731-754. (Diabetes Journals)

Delpino, F. M., et al. (2022). Ultra-processed food and risk of type 2 diabetes: A systematic review and meta-analysis. *International Journal of Epidemiology.* (PubMed)

Eisenberg, D., et al. (2022). 2022 ASMBS-IFSO guidelines on indications for metabolic and bariatric surgery. *Surgery for Obesity and Related Diseases.* (PMC)

Fothergill, E., et al. (2016). Persistent metabolic adaptation 6 years after "The Biggest Loser" competition. *Obesity, 24*(8), 1612-1619. (PMC)

Gabel, K., et al. (2019). Differential effects of alternate-day fasting versus daily calorie restriction on insulin resistance in adults with overweight or obesity and insulin resistance. *Obesity.* (PMC)

Greenwood, D. C., et al. (2013). Glycemic index, glycemic load, and risk of type 2 diabetes: A systematic review and dose-response meta-analysis. *Diabetes Care.* (PubMed)

Jackness, C., et al. (2013). Very low-calorie diet mimics the early beneficial effect of Roux-en-Y gastric bypass on insulin sensitivity and β-cell function in type 2 diabetic patients. *Diabetes, 62*(9), 3027-3032. (PMC)

Joslin, E. P. (1916). The treatment of diabetes mellitus. *Canadian Medical Association Journal, 6*(8), 673-684. (PubMed)

Malik, V. S., Popkin, B. M., Bray, G. A., Després, J. P., & Hu, F. B. (2010). Sugar-sweetened beverages and risk of metabolic syndrome and type 2 diabetes. *Diabetes Care, 33*(11), 2477-2483. (Diabetes Journals)

Mazur, A. (2011). Why were "starvation diets" promoted for diabetes in the pre-insulin period? *Nutrition Journal, 10*, 23. (PMC)

Meira, I., et al. (2024). Diabetes remission after bariatric surgery: A 10-year follow-up study. (PMC)

Pérez-Pevida, B., et al. (2019). Mechanisms underlying type 2 diabetes remission after metabolic surgery. (PMC)

Stanhope, K. L., et al. (2009). Consuming fructose-sweetened, not glucose-sweetened, beverages increases visceral adiposity and lipids and decreases insulin sensitivity in overweight/obese humans. *The Journal of Clinical Investigation, 119*(5), 1322-1334. (JCI)

World Health Organization. (2015). *Guideline: Sugars intake for adults and children.* (NCBI)

Estruch, R., Ros, E., Salas-Salvadó, J., Covas, M. I., Corella, D., Arós, F., et al. (2018). Primary prevention of cardiovascular disease with a Mediterranean diet supplemented with extra-virgin olive oil or nuts. *New England Journal of Medicine.* (New England Journal of Medicine)

Hall, K. D., Ayuketah, A., Brychta, R., Cai, H., Cassimatis, T., Chen, K. Y., et al. (2019). Ultra-processed diets cause excess calorie intake and weight gain: An inpatient randomized controlled trial. *Cell Metabolism.* (PubMed)

Lindeberg, S., Berntorp, E., Nilsson-Ehle, P., Terént, A., & Vessby, B. (1999). Low serum insulin in traditional Pacific Islanders: The Kitava study. *European Journal of Internal Medicine.* (PubMed)

Palomar-Cros, A., et al. (2023). Associations of meal timing and eating occasions with incidence of type 2 diabetes. *International Journal of Epidemiology.* (PubMed)

Salas-Salvadó, J., Bulló, M., Babio, N., Martínez-González, M. A., Ibarrola-Jurado, N., Basora, J., et al. (2011). Reduction in the incidence of type 2 diabetes with the Mediterranean diet: Results of the PREDIMED-Reus nutrition intervention randomized trial. *Diabetes Care.* (PubMed)

ISGlobal. (2023). An early breakfast may reduce the risk of developing type 2 diabetes. (ISGLOBAL)